The Program for

BETTER

VISION

The Program for
BETTER VISION

HOW TO SEE BETTER
IN MINUTES A DAY

WITHOUT GLASSES OR CONTACTS!

Martin Sussman

North Atlantic Books
Berkeley, California
Cambridge Institute for Better Vision
Topsfield, Massachusetts

The Program for Better Vision

Published by
Cambridge Institute for Better Vision
65 Wenham Road
Topsfield MA 01983

Distributed by
North Atlantic Books
P.O. Box 12327
Berkeley, California 94712

Cover design by Carole Allen

Printed in the United States of America

The Program for Better Vision is sponsored by the Society for the Study of Native Arts and Sciences, a nonprofit educational corporation whose goals are to develop an educational and cross cultural perspective linking various scientific, social, and artistic fields; to nurture a holistic view of arts, sciences, humanities, and healing; and to publish and distribute literature on the relationship of mind, body, and nature.

Library of Congress Cataloging–In–Publication Data

Sussman, Martin, 1951-
    The Program for Better Vision / Martin Sussman
        p.   cm.
    Originally published: Topsfield, Mass. : K-SEE Publications, c1995
    includes index
    ISBN 1-55643-257-7
    1. Visual training--Popular works. 2. Behavioral optometry--Popular works.   I. Title
RE960.S87   1998
617.7'5--dc21   97-38016
                                                      CIP

1 2 3 4 5 6 7 8 / 00 99 98

THOUSANDS OF PEOPLE ARE SEEING BETTER TODAY BECAUSE THEY'VE USED THE SAME TECHNIQUES THAT YOU'LL FIND IN THIS BOOK.

READ WHAT SOME HAVE TO SAY...

Plays church organ without glasses:

"For the last two years, I've been using reading glasses for everything. I play the organ at my church and I always needed my glasses for that. Once, when I forgot them, my husband had to rush in and bring them to me at the last moment.

But, deep inside, I never wanted to believe that poor vision had to be a part of aging, so I decided to start The Program for Better Vision.

The changes have been incredible. The thing that was most dramatic for me was when I took my glasses off in church and played the organ for more than two hours, reading every note perfectly with my own eyes.

I don't even need glasses to read phone numbers in the phone book. Thanks!"

Judy Washbush, Madison WI

Passes driver's test in only five weeks:

"Before I started The Program I wore my glasses 14-15 hours every single day. I passed my driver's test without them only five weeks after starting The Program. Now, I never need glasses at all. I feel much more confident and free. It's a great Program!"

Donna Sanders, Havre MT

73 years young and seeing better:

"I am 73 years old and have been wearing glasses since I was 27 — almost 50 years. I've been using The Program for just eight weeks now and already I notice improvement! I can see road signs more easily as well as smaller print on the TV. My peripheral vision is better and colors seem more vibrant and clear. I'm very excited — practice really brings results. The Program makes it easy to get improvement."

Horace Kirk, Ceres CA

Passes driver's test, reads without glasses:

"At 55 years of age, I passed my driver's test without glasses for the first time in 35 years. I no longer need glasses for reading, either. All this in about 6 to 9 months."

Albert Rioux, Jr., Manchester NH

Distance vision is better now:

"I was nearsighted and started wearing glasses when I was 17 years old. After using The Program for Better Vision I can see — without glasses — in the distance much clearer than I every could before.

When I wake up in the morning my eyesight is crystal clear. It fades a little as the day goes on, but I feel that I have already crossed a major hurdle towards clearer vision. I know that I am in control of my eyesight and I plan on continuing with The Program."

Jeffrey White, Vernon CT

Trifocals are weaker by more than 50%:

"My trifocal prescription was plus 2.25 when I started; now I read much of the time with no glasses, and when I use corrective lenses they are usually plus 1.0. If the light is poor I use plus 1.5. I wore my glasses all the waking hours before, but now only when I read and much of the time not even then. I plan to continue the program until I am completely free of corrective lenses."

Gerald N. Cox, Rapid City SD

Cole-bottle glasses are almost completely gone:

"I started wearing glasses when I was 7 or 8 years old and my vision kept deteriorating until I was very nearsighted and wearing coke-bottle-bottom glasses. (My prescription was -6.00.) Eye doctors had given up on my vision.

One year ago I started using The Program for Better Vision and now I have flashes of perfectly clear vision at times! My current vision without eyeglasses is consistently 20/60 or better. My eye doctor is absolutely astonished and amazed at my improvement. All the exercises have been helpful, particularly the affirmations, and I know I can have absolutely perfect eyesight very soon."

Frances Sgarlatti, Edgewater CO

Astigmatism disappears, nearsightedness improves, too:

"Even though I haven't been consistent in using The Program for Better Vision, I went back to my eye doctor and he told me that my astigmatism has completely disappeared and that my nearsightedness has improved too! Now, I only use my glasses for distance and for a driver's license restriction, and my eye doctor states that I am very close to getting the restriction removed. I'm so excited about my results that I plan on using The Program more regularly."

Tronnie Brassfield, Plano TX

85-year-old helps amblyopia and astigmatism:

"I now know the muscles of my eyes as well as the fingers of my hand. I am 85 years old and can focus very well and read for a long time without fatigue. Using The Program for Better Vision, I am recovered from amblyopia and astigmatism."

Aldo Mortera, Boulogne FRANCE

More relaxed and more conscious, aware:

"I saw dramatic results. I went down to a lower prescription, which I had been using six years ago. I used to feel a desperation about my vision. Now I feel hope I had never dreamed of. My vision is more relaxed and images are sharper and clearer."

Carlos Escajeda, Fabens TX

More relaxed and more conscious, aware:

"I like how my eyes feel softer and more relaxed. I am more conscious of relaxing my eyes and my mental state. This is a valuable observation. The Program is comprehensive and well thought out. I'd recommend it!"

Adrian Palmer, Salt Lake City UT

Helps vision by releasing traumatic memories:

"Thanks to your program, my eye muscles, focusing ability, eye coordination, memory, and ability to visualize have been strengthened.

Due to my strengthened ability to visualize, I had some very strong dreams. These dreams were very important because they revealed to me some events that happened early in my childhood. Due to the traumatic nature of those events, I, without knowing, blocked them from my memory.

In addition, I'm more relaxed, and my ability to see better has improved greatly. My eye doctor tested my vision and it has improved by 25% in just two months."

D.W., Atlantic City NJ

Reduces use of glasses, holds reading material further away:

"When I first started The Program, I wore my glasses all the time. After the first 8 weeks, I was able to reduce my wearing time to 8 hours a day.

My vision is improving and my eyes feel so much better. I can now hold the reading material farther away and still see clearly. I feel that if my improvement so far is any indication, I have every reason to continue The Program."

Nita Gause, San Diego CA

Nun no longer needs eye drops:

"Before I used The Program, I needed eye drops several times a day and ointment at night; now my eyes are not as tired. I do not use the drops and ointment as frequently. This new concept of eyecare has brought me help and I am appreciative."

Sister M.L.W., London, Ontario, CANADA

Was 20/200, now has clear flashes:

"My eyesight was about 20/200 when I started your Program. Now my vision is much more relaxed and there are many times that I am seeing almost perfectly."

Lenaye Seigel, Chicago IL

Impresses family with changes:

"Since completing The Program, I enjoy much more color, depth perception, and delineation of patterns. I just finished my first book without glasses and without undue effort. I read on a sun deck outside - my family was very impressed."

Mardelle McClure, Lake Jackson TX

Stimulates mind, improves attitudes:

"I have experienced major improvement in my visual attitude. The Program stimulates the mind, which is the key to everything, not just clear vision. I was impressed with the tapes and with the people I spoke to at the Institute."

Lawrence Merkler, Morrisville PA

Grateful for deep healing of painful memories:

"I was pleasantly surprised and very grateful for the depth and scope of this Program. Especially the healing techniques involved, even to the healing of memories. Now I can see more clearly for longer periods of time with less strain. I intend to never, never wear glasses again."

Michele Largey, Waltham MA

Surveyor sheds reading glasses:

"I am a surveyor and have needed reading glasses to work for more than 3 years. I started The Program for Better Vision because I wanted to be able to work without glasses. I'm pleased to report that after only 3 months, I can generally survey in most daylight conditions without needing my glasses."

Chris Hoare, Lundbreck, Alberta, CANADA

Wrote this letter without glasses:

"I was surprised to discover how sharp my vision becomes from doing The Program. I've realized that it is possible to read without my glasses, and I'm even writing this without my glasses. Thank you!"

Joanne Evans Roach, Poway CA

Headaches, tension and glasses are gone:

"I don't use glasses anymore. My headaches are gone, and I've learned how to keep tension away from my eyes and to control my body with my mind. Your Program is organized well and is very effective."

Michael Brandau, Baltimore MD

Can relax eye muscles at will:

"The Vision Sessions made me feel surprisingly relaxed. I realize it when my eye muscles are tense, and now I know how to relax them. All aspects of The Program for Better Vision are excellent."

Vesta Andrews, Red Bluff CA

Passes driver's test without glasses:

"Your EYECLASSES seminar, combined with The Program for Better Vision, *did me a lot of good. I have not worn glasses for some time, and recently passed the examination for driving in New York without glasses."*

Donald Drake, Niagara Falls NY

Needs glasses less than before:

"When I first started The Program, I wore my glasses all the time. After the first 8 weeks, I was able to experience periods of clear vision and reduce my wearing time to 5 hours a day. Thank you again - this Program is a precious stepping stone for me in my rise to clearer vision."

Claire Morneau, Montreal, Quebec, CANADA

Uses weaker glasses:

"I've worn glasses since age 7. So at first I was frustrated without wearing them, but now I enjoy not wearing glasses. The Program showed me how much more beautiful we all can be and see without glasses. It did help me to get 20/40 glasses, and I'm sure that using weaker lenses had something to do with my success."

Richard Hamre, Basel, SWITZERLAND

Passes driver's test without glasses:

"I don't need glasses anymore. I passed my driver's test without them after only four months!"

Carolyn Zelenka, Topsfield MA

Eyes feel better every week:

"It's hard to believe, but I used to wake up in the morning with tired, tense eyes. Now my eyes feel better every week. I have some tools and techniques to take charge of my vision, and I don't have to passively accept limitations on my eyesight."

Robert Coddington, Eugene OR

Skips exercises, vision improves 100%:

"One year after taking off my glasses (except for driving and movies) I was re-examined by my eye doctor. My vision improved 100% and I wasn't even regular with the exercises."

Harriet Russell, Lenox MA

Sees everything better:

"After using The Program, I notice more clarity, more contrast, more depth and brighter colors, as well as more expression in my eyes. I see everything better."

Evelyn Baril, Sheridan WY

Never needs bifocals any longer:

"Even though it's tough to admit that you're 44, I wasn't convinced that I could do anything about my 'aging' eyes. But after completing your Program, I never need bifocals to see! I can read and do close work for as long as I want."

Dr. Olga Hayes, Beverly MA

Ophthalmologist astounded:

"The ophthalmologist couldn't believe what a change I had made in my vision!"

Kate Mullaney, Rochester NY

After 25 years, he passes driver's test:

"It's official! For the first time in 25 years, I passed my driver's test without my glasses, only 18 months after I started with your techniques!"

Howard Sann, Wilton CT

Wears half as strong glasses:

"My current glasses are almost half as strong as my older pair."

L. Dirksen, Pacific Grove CA

Reads without glasses at age 89:

"After only 2 months of using your Program, reading ordinary print is much easier without glasses, and sometimes it is completely clear and effortless! I'm 89 and looking forward to more changes in the future!"

H. Leon Porter, St. Cloud FL

Has metaphysical experience:

"I was amazed to discover that my brain can command my eyes to focus. One of the sessions is a beautiful metaphysical experience for me. I find the exercises bring me new answers and insight every time I do them. Thank you for your Program and all it has meant to me."

Stephanie Collins, Las Vegas NV

Has perfect vision now:

"I went from wearing glasses all the time to tested 20/20 vision."

Pat Boll, Hartford CT

"The eyes are the windows of the soul."
– Du Bartas, Divine Weekes and Workes

"If the eyes are the windows of the soul, why are so many people wearing glasses?"
– anonymous

Dedicated to my father,
Leonard Sussman,
who was the first to introduce me to natural vision improvement.

ACKNOWLEDGMENTS

Many thanks and appreciation also go to: Heidi Neumann, for tape transcription; Roger Barnaby, the photographer; Janet Parker and Judy Kempa, illustrators; Jo Corro, the model; Behavioral optometrists Drs. Dale Freeberg and Carl Gruning for their professional advice and knowledge, Dr. Allan H. Verter, for the section on posture and to Drs. Gary Price Todd, Ben Lane, Richard Kavner and David Kubicek for their assistance on the chapter, **The Role of Nutrition in Vision**.

And to Howard Sann, who helped organize and edit the written materials that accompany the audiotape version of **The Program for Better Vision**, which was created before this book and provided the core information in it. Thanks, Howie, for hanging in there through the years.

PREFACE

I first became interested in improving my vision at 13 when my father gave me the book, *"Better Eyesight Without Glasses"* by Dr. William Bates. I had already been wearing glasses since I was nine and didn't like them, so I was willing to give it a try.

My first experiment with better vision didn't last very long. I gave up on the exercises from the book and I was soon back to getting stronger and stronger glasses.

When I was 26, I was ready to begin a more in-depth exploration of my vision. A major turning point came when I was Palming, trying to relax my eyes. I had done this exercise many times before with no apparent immediate success, but this time was different. Before I took by hands from my eyes, I suddenly felt and knew — with complete inner certainty — that I could see. When I opened my eyes, everything was clear, I really could see! (For details on how to Palm, see P. 78.)

This spell, or flash, of completely clear vision lasted for nearly 3 minutes. Though it faded and my old way of seeing at that time returned, this experience showed me that there was nothing wrong with my eyes. I really didn't even need to improve my vision, I just needed to re-awaken my ability to see and allow it to re-emerge.

I continued to explore ways to encourage this re-awakening and I continued to see better and better.

A few years later I met a dear friend, Tom Boyer, and together we began teaching others what we were learning for ourselves. We created EYECLASSES, the weekend vision seminar.

From 1977 to 1986, I traveled throughout the United States and Canada, teaching the thousands of people who participated in the EYECLASSES Seminar and seeing what worked to help them gain the most changes in their vision. I was refining what I knew had helped me and molding it into a comprehensive system that was helping others. (By now, Tom had moved on to other ventures.)

In 1985, I distilled the essence of the seminar into a home-study method using audiotapes, charts and instructional materials. This became the original Program for Better Vision.

In the 10 years since then, more than 150,000 people from around the world have asked the Cambridge Institute for help in gaining better vision. I've appeared on numerous radio and TV shows discussing natural vision care, created advanced programs and have co-written a book on computer safety, **Total Health at the Computer**.

I've received many requests from people asking me to write a comprehensive book outlining my vision improvement system that would also include new information and techniques.

You hold that book in your hands. Welcome to natural vision care.

I hope that you enjoy your process of re-awakening as much as I have!

Martin Sussman

TABLE OF CONTENTS

INTRODUCTION

CHAPTER ONE

BEFORE YOU BEGIN

If you can read this without your glasses or contact lenses take them off. But wait a second! Even if you cannot read this without your glasses or contacts, take them off for a moment. Now look around. Notice what you can see, what you cannot see and what you wish you could see.

It's natural to compare your vision without glasses to how things look with them — but don't. It's not an accurate comparison, it's not healthy and it won't produce anything positive. In fact, without the proper attitude and perspective it can only lead to frustration and to a sense of always falling short. This book will assist you to change your attitude and outlook toward your vision.

The Program also seeks to awaken your innate ability to see. Most of us have spent part of our lives not needing glasses. For some it was only the first few years; others have had clear vision well into middle age. In both cases almost all of us have demonstrated that somewhere within lies the ability to see more clearly than we do now.

Improving your vision can be exhilarating and rewarding. By deciding to use **The Program for Better Vision** you have taken your first and perhaps most significant step — the commitment to do something good about your vision.

At first the changes you notice will be in the physical aspect of your sight — less eye fatigue, less eyestrain, increased relaxation and a greater ease of seeing. And you may find that your attitudes about your self, your vision and your glasses may also begin to change. More profound changes will very likely follow as you go along.

With natural clear vision the world takes on a different sense of brightness and dimensionality — a realness that is hard to describe. Clear vision results from a relaxed mind, a healthy and vital body and a balanced emotional state.

Your active total involvement in The Program is needed to achieve the maximum results with your vision. More than a compilation of "eye exercises" to be practiced in a mechanical way, **The Program for Better Vision** is a process of self discovery, learning and growth.

Improving your eyesight is a journey involving your mind, body, emotions and spirit. You will also have the opportunity to broaden your perspective, improve your self-image, gain emotional clarity and focus your energy and concentration more effectively.

Welcome!

CHAPTER TWO

HOW TO USE THIS BOOK

To get the most benefit from this book and to achieve the most results that you can, implement these seven steps:

1. **READ** through this book once to acquire a general overview.

2. **DECIDE** what glasses/contact lenses to use and how to use them while improving your vision. (Pp. 54 - 56)

3. **SET UP** your practice area. (Pp. 57 - 58)

4. **CHOOSE** a practice time.

5. **START** and **COMPLETE** THE FIRST STAGE 8-week schedule. (Pp. 106 - 121)

6. **MAIL** THE FIRST STAGE Report (Parts A - C) to the Cambridge Institute when you finish THE FIRST STAGE 8-week schedule. (Pp. 195 - 198)

7. **CONTINUE** to improve your vision. See THE SECOND STAGE for steps you can take after the initial 8-week schedule. (Pp. 125 - 126)

If you have any questions about anything contained in this book, feel free to call the Cambridge Institute's Support Line (508-887-3883) or write: 65 Wenham Road, Dept. BK-1, Topsfield MA 01983.

CHAPTER THREE

BETTER VISION IS MORE THAN 20/20

The eyes do not exist in isolation. They are an integral part of your total being affected by — and affecting — the body, mind and emotions in a profound way.

All parts of the visual system — the eyes, the muscles around and in the eyes, the nerve pathways to the brain and the visual centers of the brain — are very delicate and require a high degree of precision, coordination and flexibility to perform optimally. Since it is such a delicate system it is very sensitive to stress, tension and fatigue of any kind, whether it's physical, emotional or mental. The visual system is also very sensitive to any nutritional deficiencies and imbalances that might be present in the body.

A holistic model of **Better Vision** includes these three components:

1. Physical eyesight
2. Inner vision
3. Emotional seeing

1. Physical eyesight involves more than just 20/20 vision. In fact, there are three major visual skills:

First, your mind selects what it wants to see from its total field of vision. **(SKILL ONE: Peripheral Awareness and Central/Peripheral Balance)**

Second, your mind commands the eyes to look at or to converge on the object. **(SKILL TWO: Convergence/Binocularity)**

Third, your eyes bring the object into focus to see it clearly. **(SKILL THREE: Accommodation/Focusing)**

In addition, the muscles in and around the eyes must be relaxed, toned and flexible.

Tension, stress and imbalance in any of the three visual skills can lead to other visual difficulties in addition to focusing problems. Some of these difficulties might include: eyestrain and fatigue, headaches, glasses and contacts never feeling right, difficulty concentrating, poor eye-hand coordination and depth perception and eyes always feeling tired.

2. Inner vision is the Mind's Eye in all its different aspects: imagination, visualization, memory, dreams and attitudes. With **Better Vision** your imagination and visualization will be more alive and vivid and your memory will become clearer. Your attitudes about yourself and others will become more positive. You will replace limiting images of yourself with a clearer and more positive sense of who you are.

3. Emotional seeing speaks about our recognition of the eyes as both a way to express how we feel and a way to connect to other people. The eyes are so often called "the windows of the soul"; **Better Vision** is a way to heal, clarify and open these windows, allowing us to be open to a deeper connection to others and to give and receive more easily and fully.

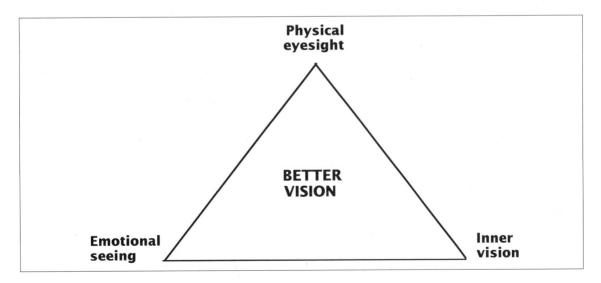

Vision problems often appear when there is both prolonged stress in the visual system and improper visual/muscular habit patterns. Nearsightedness, farsightedness and astigmatism are some of the symptoms that result from this underlying tension and imbalance.

Glasses and contacts treat the symptoms of poor vision very effectively: when you put them on you temporarily get rid of poor vision.

But glasses and contacts do not address the underlying factors that produced the vision problem. They do nothing to release the underlying stress or change the underlying patterns that caused the problem in the first place.

In addition to the issues discussed in **How The Eyes Work** (Pp. 16 - 19) physical eyesight is influenced by three other factors:

1. **Secondary tension** that is stored in other areas of the body. Also, the overall health and nutritional level of the body also affects vision. (See **Your Body and Your Eyes** [Pp. 20 23] and **The Role of Nutrition in Vision** [Pp. 24 - 37]).

2. **Limiting or negative thoughts** about vision or about how external reality is perceived . (See **Your Mind and Your Eyes** (Pp. 38 - 43).

3. **Subconscious memories and past emotional decisions**. (See **Your Emotions and Your Eyes** (Pp. 44 - 48).

All these factors influence each person in a different way and to a different degree. But in following a holistic approach to improving your vision, it is important to explore what effect each may have had on your eyesight.

According to a holistic model, **Better Vision** means seeing the world in the clearest, most relaxed, easiest and most efficient way possible. **Better Vision** also means having a positive image of yourself, a clear sense of purpose and emotional clarity.

CHAPTER FOUR

WHAT TO EXPECT

The Program for Better Vision is easy to use and will take you step by step on the road to **Better Vision**.

The goal of **The Program for Better Vision** is to improve your sight to its most natural, balanced and clearest state — thereby reducing, eliminating or postponing the use of glasses or contact lenses. Another goal of The Program is to assist you in opening your vision on the deeper levels as well — seeing with more clarity who you are, where you are going and how you relate to others.

Also, **The Program for Better Vision** will help you address the different levels that may be affecting your vision. The Program helps you bring your Physical eyesight, your Emotional seeing and your Inner vision into greater balance and harmony.

You will also learn how to:
- Relax your eyes and lessen visual stress
- Create and promote healthy visual habits
- Enhance your understanding of your vision — how it works and what factors influence it
- Heighten and maintain your visual awareness.

The most common symptoms of visual imbalance and tension are nearsightedness, farsightedness, astigmatism and difference between the eyes. Most often, these symptoms are merely the tip of the iceberg. For improvement to occur, the underlying factors that produced these symptoms must be addressed first.

Each person is different — how fast and how much a person improves is an individual matter. Even two people who have the same problem to the same degree could very well improve at different speeds and to different levels. This disparity exists for two reasons: 1) Poor vision can be caused by a variety of factors that influence each person differently ; 2) Gaining **Better Vision** is an art, not a science. Changing habit patterns comes easier to some people than to others. Learning how to relax is easier for some. Changing how you use your eyes cannot really be "taught", but is a learning that can only come through direct experience.

The purpose of the initial 8-week schedule of **The First Stage** is to balance and improve the crucial skills mentioned above. It also helps to open the brain/eye connection and release the emotional stress and mental tension that limit vision.

Within the initial 8-week period, many people see a 10 to 50% improvement. Greater results can follow after that for those who continue working on their vision. Some reach the point where they no longer need any corrective lenses. Others reach the point where they use glasses that are much, much weaker than the ones they needed when they started **The Program**.

As these underlying factors are successfully addressed it may then be appropriate to focus specific attention on your symptoms. That is why we make **The Second Stage** available to you.

We suggest that a person continue practicing until the time comes that they do not experience **any** changes in vision for at least 30 - 45 days. Some people hit this plateau soon; others reach it after two years and some are still improving years after they first begin.

No matter how "bad" your vision may be now — you can train yourself to have **Better Vision**. And, by doing something good for your eyes today you are probably preventing future, even more serious, problems from developing.

Ultimately, the amount of improvement you get is up to you. Your desire and motivation, your inner willingness to change and the time and effort you put into this journey are the personal keys that will determine your degree of success.

PART 1

YOU
AND
YOUR VISION

CHAPTER FIVE

THE FIVE COMMON MISCONCEPTIONS

Many people — even if they would like to see without corrective lenses — are skeptical that it's possible.

Much of that skepticism is rooted in misunderstanding. There are five common misconceptions that lead people to think that eyesight cannot be improved. They are:

1. Poor vision is inherited.
2. Vision inevitably deteriorates with age.
3. Poor vision is caused by certain visual activities.
4. Weak eye muscles cause poor vision.
5. Seeing is solely a physical, mechanical process.

Let's examine each of these in greater detail.

1. Poor vision is inherited

The first misconception is that vision problems are inherited; that is, if your parents had poor vision, then you will too. Once universally accepted, it is now recognized by most eye doctors that the ability to see is not fixed at birth.

Only 3 people out of every 100 who cannot see clearly are born with inherited vision problems. The other 97% develop vision problems at some point in their life. Just as we learn how to talk or how to walk, we also learn how to see.

Since most of us were actually born with clear vision it would be more accurate to say that we learned how to **not** see clearly. Of course, we didn't learn it deliberately or consciously, and we weren't taught it by anyone, but we did develop an improper way of using our eyes and brain that led to unclear vision.

Recent studies indicate that even 1-day old babies can focus clearly. When shown a picture of their mothers' face, these little infants could bring the picture into focus by adjusting the rate of their sucking on an artificial nipple. If they sucked at the right rate, the picture would stay clear. If they sucked too fast or too slow, the picture went out of focus. Invariably, the infants were able to keep the picture in focus!

Until this ingenious experiment was conducted, scientists erroneously thought that babies couldn't focus clearly until 3 or 4 months of age. Instead, it turns out that it was the scientists' inability to communicate with babies that led to their misunderstanding.

As human beings, we learn about the world around us through our five physical senses. The most dominant and highly developed is vision. In fact, 80 to 90% of the information that we gather comes to us through our eyes. Our vision is our primary means of relationship to the world around us.

Over half the people in this country wear glasses or contacts. Needing corrective lenses to see clearly is now considered normal. We have become a nation of people largely dependent on an artificial means to perform a most basic and essential human function.

Yet, it wasn't always this way. Vision problems affect five times as many people today as compared to 100 years ago. This huge increase took place during only three or four generations. If poor vision was inherited, who could we have possibly inherited it from?

2. Vision inevitably deteriorates with age

The second misconception is that vision inevitably deteriorates with age, and that everyone will eventually need glasses for reading.

The visual system — just like any other part of your body — can deteriorate with age. This is certainly true if nothing is done to retain its inherit youthfulness and flexibility, and if years of accumulated tension and rigidity are not released. But this decline is not inevitable and it is not irreversible. In fact, nothing is further from the truth.

As just one example, The Cambridge Institute recently received a letter from a remarkable 89-year-old man who had been using the same vision improvement system that you are about to start. He said in his letter, "I had been wearing reading glasses for 50 years, since I was 39. Now after 2 months of using **The Program for Better Vision** there are times when I can read without my glasses and it's completely clear and effortless."

That's a pretty amazing change, but the part of the letter that was the most striking was when he said, "I learned that I can succeed in helping myself and I'm looking forward to more changes in the future." Now, that's a youthful attitude!

Your eyes and your visual system respond to exercise, relaxation and stress relief. It all depends on the attitude you have and the concrete steps that you take to retain the vision that you have.

In fact it is our experience that middle-aged sight (presbyopia) responds very quickly to training. Many people who start to use **The Program** are able to not only halt the decline of their vision but also return it to its former degree of clarity.

3. Poor vision is caused by certain visual activities

The third misconception is that poor vision is caused by what you do with your eyes: if you read too much, or use a computer, or watch too much TV, it will ruin your eyes.

And statistics *seem* to point in that direction:

Only 2% of students in the fourth grade are nearsighted; in the 8th grade, about 10 - 20% are; by the end of college between 50 and 70% of the students are nearsighted. Thus, it would seem that the more you read or study, the more likely it would be that you would become nearsighted.

But it is not because of the activity. It is because of **how** the eyes are used when performing the activity. And nobody is ever taught how to properly use their eyes and how to protect the good vision that they were born with.

When people are taught how to properly use and rest their eyes, then vision problems are much less prevalent.

For example, in China, students and workers are taught simple eye exercises that they practice every day in school and in the factory. And the rate of nearsightedness (myopia) has decreased substantially.

Unfortunately, these techniques are not yet common practice in this country. But there have been a handful of school systems that have incorporated these and other changes with just as promising results as in China.

Extended periods of study, reading and computer use place added nutritional demands on the eyes and the body which, if not adequately met, can also contribute to visual difficulties. (See **The Role of Nutrition in Vision**, Pp. 24 - 37.)

But, there is no question that it is the visual *habits* that are critical, not the visual *activity*. The real problem is a lack of education. Vision care principles need to become more widely known and accepted, and more widely practiced.

Someday, there will be such a shift in attitude in this country. But you don't have to wait. Right now you can do something good for your eyes and protect your eyesight by practicing the right way to use your eyes. (See **10 Habits for Better Vision,** Pp. 158 - 165.)

4. Weak eye muscles cause poor vision

The fourth misconception is that weak eye muscles cause poor vision.

Yet, the muscles around the eyes are 150 to 200 times stronger than they need to be for normal use. These muscles rarely weaken. Instead, tension builds up and affects these muscles, preventing them from moving in a natural, fluid manner — their movements become stiff and restricted.

An analogy: If a person is right handed, the muscles on the right side of the body will be stronger — and more coordinated — than those on the left. Why? Only because they have been used more, not because they are inherently weaker.

The same is true for eye muscles: Over time, certain visual patterns and habits develop, and some eye muscles become stronger and more coordinated than others. But the primary source of the problem is the underlying patterns and habits. And the eyes can be trained to function with new, more effective patterns. As this retraining occurs, the symptoms of visual difficulties — such as nearsightedness, farsightedness, etc. — decrease and disappear.

5. Seeing is solely a physical, mechanical process

The fifth misconception is that seeing is a mechanical process and that clear vision is determined only by the shape of the eye. If the eye is the correct shape, the result is clear vision; if it is misshapen or distorted the result is nearsightedness, farsightedness or astigmatism.

Actually, the shape of the eye is one element in the visual system, but not the only one. (See the next chapter, **How The Eyes Work**.) As just one example, eye doctors have long known that even though two people have exactly the same refractive error (how far from the retina the distorted image registers), each could have a completely different measurement of acuity (how clearly they can read the test letters on the eye chart.) Mechanical measurement alone does not exactly predict how much a person can see. Other factors besides the shape of the eye are involved.

Many people notice that they see better at some times during the day than others. Some notice decreased vision when tired or under stress. What accounts for these daily fluctuations?

Have you ever driven down the highway, so engrossed in your thoughts and daydreams that you don't "see" your exit? Or been so tired that you read page after page without understanding a word?

Vision is a dynamic, changing process, affected by many different physical, emotional and mental factors. The shape of the eye may be one factor, but even that can change as a result of training and nutrition.

Let's look at how the eyes work, and the roles played by the body, mind and emotions in vision. Once we gain a fuller understanding of the holistic nature of vision, we'll be ready to see better for ourselves.

CHAPTER SIX

HOW THE EYES WORK

The working of the eyes is often compared to the way a camera operates. Let's look at that analogy, and see where it holds true and where it breaks down.

The camera has a lens to focus the light, a way to control the focusing, a shutter to let in the desired amount of light, and film that holds the image.

The eye has a lens, a focusing mechanism (controlled by the ciliary muscles), an iris (which adjusts the amount of light entering the eye through the pupil), and a retina (where the image is recorded). (Fig. 1)

In a camera, for the image to be clear it must be focused on the film. Likewise, in the eye, the image must be focused on the retina (film). (Fig. 2A)

In a nearsighted eye, rather than the image registering precisely on the retina, it is focused in front of the retina. (Fig. 2B) Thus, one conclusion is that the eyeball is too long. In a farsighted eye, the opposite happens: The image is focused behind the retina. (Fig. 2C) Here, the conclusion is that the eyeball is too short.

If these conclusions are true, how did the eyeball lose its natural shape?

There are six muscles that surround each eye and control eye movements (Fig. 3). They move your eyes up, down, to the right and to the left. When you look at something up close they turn the eyes in (converge) and when you look at a distant object they turn the eyes out (diverge). These extra-ocular muscles are 150 - 200 times stronger than they need to be. Tension in these muscles causes eye movements to become more rigid and less flexible.

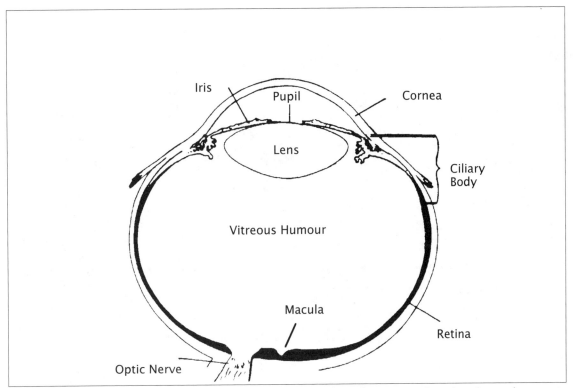

Fig. 1   The working of the eye has been compared to that of a camera, but there's much more to vision than that.

In 1981, research performed by Peter Greene at Harvard University showed that when these muscles hold the eyes in one position for an extended period of time, they also squeeze the eye. And, that under the right conditions, this pressure can change the shape of the eye.

But this is not the whole story.

Let's return to the camera analogy for a moment. In the camera, the lens moves in and out to bring objects at different distances into focus. This doesn't happen in your eyes. Instead, the lens changes its shape to bring objects into focus. (Fig. 4)

When focusing on a near object, the lens becomes fatter, bulging from front to back (Fig. 4b). To focus on something farther away, it becomes thinner (Fig. 4c). We are always changing what we are looking at, so the lens is continually making fine adjustments in its shape. Normally, the lens changes its shape — and its focus — more than 100,000 times every day.

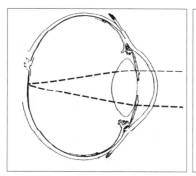

Fig. 2A To be clear, the image must be focused directly on the retina.

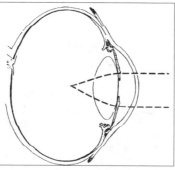

Fig. 2B The nearsighted eye brings the image to focus IN FRONT OF the retina.

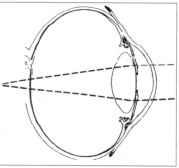

Fig. 2C The farsighted eye brings the image to focus BEHIND the retina.

The shape of the lens, and thus its focusing ability, is controlled by the ciliary body, which surrounds the lens. There is a constant and delicate interplay among the muscles and ligaments of the ciliary body. They work together to change the lens into the exact shape required to bring whatever you are looking at into sharp focus.

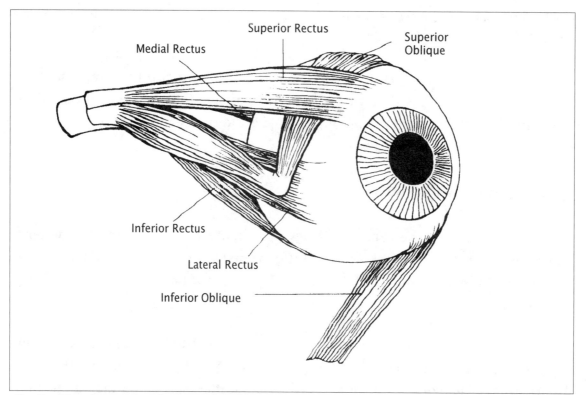

Fig. 3   The six muscles that encircle each eye are 150-200 times stronger than they need to be for normal usage.

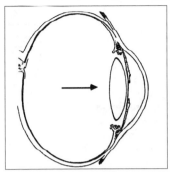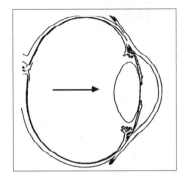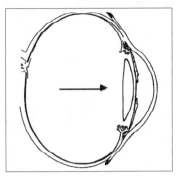

Fig. 4   The lens changes shape to bring objects at different distances into focus on the retina, bulging to bring near objects into focus (4B) and flattening to bring distant objects into focus (4C).

In the normal eye, the muscles are constantly readjusting their pull on the lens — changing the focusing power by changing its shape. The muscles and the lens are flexible, and are able to adjust and re-adjust to bring objects at near or far distance into clear focus. This process is called accommodation.

The nearsighted eye can see near objects clearly, but not distant objects. It is "stuck" for near vision, changing its shape only enough to bring near objects into focus. ***To see distant objects more clearly*** the lens needs to flatten (become thinner) to bring distant objects into sharper focus.

The farsighted eye can see distant objects clearly, but not near ones. It is "stuck" for distance vision, changing its shape only enough to bring distant objects into focus. ***To see near objects more clearly*** the lens needs to become thicker to bring nearer objects into sharper focus.

If the image isn't focused on the retina, it could be due to a decreased flexibility of the ciliary body, not a distorted shape of the eye. In fact, the lens has such a great range of focusing ability that it could easily compensate for any supposedly abnormal shape that the eye may have become.

Clear vision isn't only determined by the strength of the eye muscles. And it isn't just a matter of the shape of the eye. Instead, clear vision requires that all parts of the visual system — ciliary body, lens, extra-ocular muscles, shape of the eye — work together and function in harmony with flexibility and coordination.

And this coordination is ultimately a reflection of how the mind controls the eyes — which can be changed and retrained.

CHAPTER SEVEN

YOUR BODY AND YOUR EYES

Learning how to use the body properly and how to develop proper posture will go a long way towards promoting better vision.

Vision can be affected by tension that exists anywhere in the body, but secondary physical tension has the most profound effect on eyesight. Secondary physical tension is body tension — usually localized in the chest, shoulders, neck, head, face and jaw — that limits the free movement and functioning of the eyes.

Recent studies show that postural imbalances are almost always connected to poor vision. This is particularly true in the case of astigmatism but applies almost equally to nearsightedness, farsightedness, crossed eyes and lazy eye. Interestingly, different patterns of secondary tension are associated with different eye problems.

For example, nearsighted people often hold tension in their upper back, shoulders, base of the neck and around the eyes.

On the other hand, farsighted people tend to experience more tension in the front part of the upper body — the chest, throat and jaw areas.

People with astigmatism are more prone to exhibit twists and imbalances in their posture — as if the distortion of the eye is mirrored in the body.

And those people who have a lack of eye coordination or who see differently out of each eye also mirror that in the body. Poor eye-hand coordination and a poor sense of balance are common symptoms.

Everything that a person does to relax and to improve health will have a positive effect on eyesight. Particularly beneficial is aerobic activity, which increases the circulation and oxygen supply to the upper body.

Posture and vision

Correct posture plays a vital role in facilitating the flow of blood to and from the head, brain and visual system. In fact, as much as one third of all the blood that goes to the head nourishes the visual system.

Dr. Allan H. Verter, a Nutley, New Jersey chiropractor who helps people eliminate stress through diet, exercise and attitude, believes good posture is fairly simple to gain and maintain. "Good posture," he says, "should feel comfortable, natural and energizing — not stiff or tiring."

First attempts at changing your postural habits may feel a little "awkward or even difficult," he says, since "we've spent most of our lives sitting, standing and lying down improperly. These newer and better habits will soon become easy and second nature."

The spine's job

The spine bears the main responsibility for holding the trunk, neck and head upright. It has its own supporting foundation in the pelvis and lower extremities and receives assistance from the rib cage.

The single most important rule of correct posture is to hold the spine in a comfortable straight line at normal full height without any sagging or slouching. This is accomplished by having each of the 24 vertebrae (which make up the spinal column) move or push away from each other until there is no sag or slouch left in the ligaments and muscles connecting them. The shoulders and rib cage should always stay relaxed, whether you are sitting or standing.

Sitting

When sitting always have all or at least some portion of your pelvis (buttocks) all the way back in your seat so that it is making contact with the back of the chair. If there is a problem with your feet reaching the floor and you cannot adjust the chair height, use a firm pillow to fill in the gap between your buttocks and the chair back. (Fig. 5)

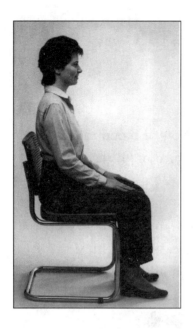

Fig. 5   Sitting in a relaxed and balanced manner contributes to better vision. Sit with your pelvis back in the seat and your feet touching the floor. Do not slouch, sag or curve your shoulders in. Let your weight rest on your pelvis.

Avoid letting your pelvis slide forward (slouching) or dropping your mid-back against the chair back. With your pelvis in contact with the chair back, it's okay to lean your trunk (from the waist up) forward and away from it — as long as your spine and trunk do not sag or slouch.

Last, your arms must not be used to hold the trunk and body upright. They may rest on a desk, the arms of a chair or be used to hold down papers, etc., but from the waist up your body should maintain itself in an upright position under its own power (again without slouching).

Standing

When standing upright let your body weight distribute itself equally forward, backward, and to the right and left sides around your spine. Think of a column of children's building blocks. If any block is placed too far forward, backward or to either side, the column will become unstable and topple. Keeping your weight evenly distributed at all levels avoids creating any toppling, tilting or tipping stresses (or strains) on your spine and the rest of your skeletal system.

You might look at yourself in a mirror from both the front and side positions to help see if you have acquired any postural imbalances. If you have any, gently guide the tipped or tilted areas (such as the pelvis, trunk, abdomen, head or shoulders) back into a position of natural balance. This includes making sure that your weight is evenly distributed in both feet. In a short time, you will be able to correct your own posture without using a mirror.

Lying down and neck support

When lying on your back or side use pillow support for your head and neck. Tuck some of the pillow under the back or side of your neck to support the normally forward curve of your cervical spine, (which gravity would otherwise cause to straighten as you recline). Don't overdo this support under the neck. Roll or tuck the lower third or quarter of the pillow under the back or side of your neck (depending on whether you are lying on your back or side). The rest of the pillow can lie under your head.

If you lie on your side often, it is best to alternate lying on either side rather than favoring one. This will relieve the spine of always being subject to the pull of gravity from only one side.

Reading and TV

People with vision difficulties should only watch TV and read while sitting upright. Lying down while engaged in these activities places unneeded distortion and stress on the visual system.

CHAPTER EIGHT

THE ROLE OF NUTRITION IN VISION

The visual system — the eyes, muscles, nerves and vision centers of the brain — is one of the most complex and highly demanding systems of the body.

More than 25% of the nutrition your body absorbs goes to feed the visual system. The visual system consumes one third of all the oxygen that you take in. Metabolism in the eyes is faster than anywhere else in the body. The concentration of vitamin C in the healthy eye is higher than almost anywhere else in the body.

It's not surprising, then, that proper nutrition plays an extremely important role in preventing and treating all of the common eye problems — myopia, presbyopia, cataract, glaucoma and macular degeneration. Nutrition's exact role is becoming more and more clear. Some facts are already well documented and pioneering doctors are uncovering other directions that are very promising.

Before we can discuss each eye problem in greater detail, it's important to keep in mind some general nutritional information:

1. Proper balance is important. The body does not use each vitamin and mineral in isolation. The absence of one may affect the body's ability to use another. For example, proper amounts of magnesium and vitamin D are needed in order to absorb calcium efficiently and completely. And, without adequate levels of zinc, the body cannot utilize all the vitamin A it receives.

2. Minimum Daily Requirements (MDR) recommended by the United States government are just that — minimum levels. Visual health most probably requires supplement levels that are significantly higher than the minimum. Cataract

prevention, for example, may require the intake of vitamin C at a level 15 times greater than the minimum daily requirement.

3. In today's society, it is probably not realistic to expect to get all of our nutrients from food alone. No matter how wholesome and pure our diet might be, there are other factors that affect the nutrient content of the food we eat. How food is grown, how it is stored and how it is cooked all affect its nutrient value. Besides, the amount of nutrients a particular food is *supposed* to contain is measured under ideal laboratory conditions, which probably don't reflect the food you are actually eating. Most of us have long known that carrots and vitamin A are supposed to be good for the eyes. Even so, 68% of the population is deficient in vitamin A.

4. On the other hand, "popping" vitamin pills is no substitute for a wholesome diet. The body loses a significant amount of nutrients depending on the kind of food we consume. For example, we lose the trace mineral chromium as our body tries to absorb white sugar. And caffeine, refined flour, medication and preservatives also leach trace minerals and vitamins from our system. Also, there may be as yet undiscovered vitamins and minerals in food that someday will prove to be very important to our health.

5. Age, activity level and stress affect what your body needs and how well your body can absorb and use what nutrients it does get.

Keeping these general ideas in mind, let's look at the role that nutrition may play in various eye conditions.

Myopia

Myopia (nearsightedness) is a condition that affects nearly 1 out of every 3 people in the United States. Yet, only 3 out of every 100 myopic people are born that way; for everyone else, myopia is acquired at some point during their life span.

Myopia is the result of a degeneration of some part of the visual system. It's so common to see someone wearing glasses that we forget that it is not natural. Myopic people are also more prone to develop more serious eye conditions, such as retinal detachment, glaucoma and cataracts.

The search for nutritional answers to myopia has focused on two different parts of the visual system: the shape of the eye and the functioning of the lens.

Let's look at each of these separately:

One possible explanation for myopia is that it occurs when the eye elongates, stretching from front to back (Fig. 2B, P. 18). Distortions as small as 4/100 of an inch are enough to produce extreme degrees of myopia. Exactly what causes this stretching is not clear, though it seems to be due to either increased intraocular pressure or excessive tension in the extra-ocular muscles.

Dr. Gary Price Todd, a North Carolina ophthalmologist, has been using nutritional and metabolic healing for different eye problems for more than 20 years. He is trained to do all the standard surgeries for the eyes, but he prefers to promote the natural healing of the eyes whenever possible.

Dr. Todd believes that most myopia develops in children during growth spurts. If the child is not receiving proper nutrition, the body literally takes minerals from the eye to use in the growth of the body. The resulting mineral depletion in the eye weakens its structure, making it susceptible to the forces and stresses involved in prolonged near work, including reading, studying, watching TV or using a computer — all of which are common activities for most of today's children.

Dr. Todd has success in arresting the progression of myopia in children that he treats; in some cases, the degree of myopia has decreased. Dr. Todd achieves these results just by recommending that children under his care supplement their diet with his basic vitamin and mineral formula, NUTRIPLEX, which is particularly rich in the minerals selenium, chromium and zinc. (See P. 201 for a listing of the ingredients in NUTRIPLEX.)

Dr. Ben Lane, New Jersey optometrist and another pioneer in the role of nutrition in myopia and other eye diseases, concurs in the importance of these trace minerals in maintaining the strength of the eye. Dr. Lane has found that chromium levels in myopic children are 1/3 that of children with normal vision. (It is interesting to note that chromium is depleted in the body by white sugar, eaten all too frequently by many children today.)

Calcium levels are also lower in nearsighted children. Dr. Lane found that children increasing in the degree of myopia have diets extremely deficient in calcium. Dr. Lane thinks that in the face of this dietary deficiency, the body takes calcium from the eye to help support bone growth. This calcium lack then makes the eye susceptible to the forces playing on it during prolonged periods of near work and visual stress. Dr. Lane has also found that these children also eat too much meat protein (a poor source of calcium) and too little calcium-rich milk products and stalky vegetables. Caffeine (found in soda as well as in coffee) is known to leach calcium from the body.

Dr. Lane has also found that Vitamin C is important. He has noted that low levels of dietary intake of Vitamin C are associated with increases in pressure in the eye. This increasing pressure also is associated with the visual fatigue that can result from extended periods of near work. The focusing mechanism needs adequate levels of vitamin C and chromium for efficient functioning. Adequate levels of Vitamin C are also needed to ensure the strength of the eyes.

Vitamin C is leached from the body by artificial flavors and ingredients and aspirin. It is generally recommended that an adult take between 500 and 1000 mg. a day, increasing the quantity during periods of high stress (including visual stress — extended periods of near range work).

Another vitamin that Dr. Lane thinks is of critical importance is folic acid, which helps the eyes to maintain near focus for longer periods of time as well as increase the eyes' ability to absorb nutrition from the body. He thinks that folic acid should come from food sources rather than from vitamins.

Drs. Todd and Lane have focused their studies on the nutritional factors involved in maintaining the structural integrity of the eye. Another explanation for myopia, also incorporated in Dr. Lane's theory, is that the lens has lost some of its ability to change focus, due to the constant pressure placed on it to maintain near point focus (e.g., when reading, writing, using a computer).

According to this theory, myopia occurs when the lens becomes "stuck" for near point vision and is unable to shift its focus to distant objects. Normally, the lens has the power to change its focus more than enough to compensate for individual differences in the length of the eye.

Dr. David A. Kubicek, a California doctor of chiropractic, explored the role of the lens in a research paper he wrote in 1988. This is a synopsis of his theory and his recommendations:

The ciliary muscle (which controls the focusing of the lens) is itself stimulated by both the sympathetic and the parasympathetic nerve systems of the body. Parasympathetic stimulation increases accommodation — the lens' ability to focus on near objects. Sympathetic stimulation decreases this ability, allowing the lens to focus on distant objects. Clear vision at all distances requires the nervous system of the body to constantly balance and re-balance these two types of stimulation.

Nearsighted people, Dr. Kubicek reasoned, would lack sufficient sympathetic stimulation to bring distant objects into focus. Farsighted people, on the other hand, would show a weakness in parasympathetic stimulation.

To test his theory, Dr. Kubicek devised a simple muscular test that would tell him which system was weak for an individual. By performing only this simple test, he was able to predict — with 100% accuracy — which subjects were nearsighted and which were farsighted. Dr. Kubicek was then able to use this procedure and his knowledge of biochemistry to devise the right combination of nutrients that could promote proper functioning of the lens and thus help to improve vision at all distances.

Certain nutrients are known to increase sympathetic activity and others are known to increase parasympathetic activity. Nutrients that might be beneficial to nearsighted people would be vitamins B-2 and B-6, folic acid, niacinamide, zinc, magnesium and phosphorus, among others. (On the other hand, Dr. Lane cautions against phosphorus intake. His research indicates that what is most important is maintaining the balance in the body between calcium and phosphorus, a balance which is upset by the intake of too much animal-derived protein.)

Dr. Kubicek has spent the last five years formulating what he considers to be exactly the right combination of these — and other — critical nutrients, and he is nearing the stage when he can make this formula available to the general public.

Presbyopia

Presbyopia is more commonly known as "middle-aged sight" — the deterioration of near vision as a person ages, with the need for reading glasses beginning at about age forty.

Presbyopia occurs when the lens loses enough of its plasticity and elasticity so that it can no longer adequately respond to the visual demand to focus at near. The lens has no blood supply of its own, receiving nutrients through the ciliary body. The lens' cells will break down when they do not receive the proper supply of nutrients. Presbyopia is one symptom of this breakdown. If the breakdown of the lens continues, the stage is set for cataract formation.

Therefore, it would seem logical that the presbyopic eye would respond to the same kind of nutritional approaches that have been shown to prevent cataract formation. In fact, Dr. Todd is finding exactly that. Patients following his nutritional treatment for cataracts are finding that their presbyopia often improves as well.

An Italian study, conducted nearly 50 years ago, found that vitamin E — an anti-oxidant critical in the prevention of cataracts — helped presbyopic people regain their near point vision. Unfortunately, other than this one study, no other nutritional research has been done on presbyopia.

Cataracts

In the United States, approximately four million people have some degree of cataracts, while 40,000 are blinded due to cataracts. One in every five people over 55 are afflicted with cataracts, and as many as half of those over 75 are at risk. Worldwide, cataracts are the leading cause of blindness.

The standard treatment for cataracts is surgery. In fact, cataract surgery is the most common of *all* surgical procedures practiced in the United States, with more than 500,000 performed each and every year.

94% of cataract surgeries are successful, with lower vision resulting in less than 6 out of every 100 procedures. It is one of the safest operation in the world, but it still has some degree of risk associated with it.

Even though the surgical treatment for cataracts is highly successful, it is an extremely costly procedure. Each cataract surgery (one eye only) done in the United States costs approximately $5,000. Every year, over 4 billion dollars are spent — just by Medicare alone! — for cataract surgery.

As people live longer and longer, the incidence of cataracts can only increase, if no preventative measures are taken. If the development of cataracts could be delayed by 10 years, the National Eye Institute estimates that half of all cataract surgery could be eliminated, saving billions of dollars every year in medical costs.

What is a cataract?

Light enters the eye through the lens. The healthy lens is completely transparent — as clear as the water in a glass — and allows light to enter unobstructed. It is also pliable and elastic so that it can respond to changes in focusing.

The lens is growing throughout life with layer upon layer of new cells growing on top of the center (nucleus) of the lens, much like the rings of a tree. Therefore the lens becomes thicker as it grows (its nucleus has the same cells it had at birth). Without protective or preventative measures, it becomes more and more difficult over time for the nucleus to receive all the nutrients that it needs.

If the breakdown in the nucleus continues, the lens becomes cloudy and loses its transparency. This is a cataract.[1]

A cataract starts out small and, if left untreated, gets larger over time, becoming thicker and thicker and covering more and more of the lens. A cataract needs to grow large enough before surgery can be performed; that's why ordinary medical advice is to sit back and wait until the cataract is large enough — "ripe" — for surgery. Fortunately, it is during this early "growing" stage that nutritional treatment can be the most successful.

---

[1] Nuclear cataract — a cataract that begins in the center (nucleus) of the lens — is the most common kind of cataract, affecting people as they age. But there are two other types as well: Anterior cortical cataract (cloudiness forms in the front of the lens) and posterior, subcapsular cataract (cloudiness forms in the back of the lens). Both of these types occur much more rarely.

There is plenty of evidence that cataracts can be prevented, and their growth arrested, with proper nutrition. According to both Drs. Lane and Todd, prevention is the key. "With the right nutritional supplements, prevention rates could be very close to 100%," says Dr. Todd.

Most research in the United States has focused on the prevention of cataracts. It is a generally accepted fact that cataracts are a degenerative disease caused by free radical damage and that they can be prevented with anti-oxidant vitamins C and E, beta carotene and some trace minerals, including selenium and chromium.

The eye has the highest concentration of vitamin C of any part of the body. Yet, lenses with cataracts have much lower levels of vitamin C than cataract-free lenses. The eye with a cataract has also been shown to be deficient in selenium, copper, manganese, zinc and glutathione (which the body normally produces on its own, but only if adequate levels of selenium are present). Some of the B vitamins — particularly niacin and riboflavin — have also been deficient in the eye with a cataract, though this deficiency is rare in the United States, where many processed foods are "enriched" with these vitamins. Excesses of mercury and other toxins have also been implicated.

According to a recent study conducted by John Hopkins University, people with the highest levels of vitamin E in their blood were 50% less likely to develop cataracts. A study reported in the Archives of Ophthalmology in 1988 showed that 200 IU a day of vitamin E reduces the incidence of cataracts by 56%. If 250 mgs. of vitamin C are added, their incidence is reduced by 86%.

Also in 1988, a Canadian study found that elderly subjects taking either 300 - 600 mg of vitamin C or 400 IU of vitamin E over a five year period were 56 - 70% less likely to develop age-related cataracts than would otherwise be predicted.

Unfortunately, there hasn't been as much research in the United States devoted to the nutritional treatment of cataracts once they develop. However, nutritional treatment of cataracts is routine in Germany, France and Japan.

In the United States, Dr. Todd has been using nutritional supplements for years to treat patients with cataracts. He finds that if nutritional treatment is started soon enough (when vision is 20/50 or better), he is nearly 100% successful in stopping its progression or reversing the cataract.

In one study conducted by Dr. Todd over a 1-year period, 43% of the people showed improvement in their cataract and the other 57% stabilized the cataract completely and showed absolutely no further deterioration. All of these results held up in a follow-up study conducted 5 years after the original. Cataract surgery was avoided in every case.

As a result of this and earlier studies, Dr. Todd has created a complete vitamin and mineral formula different from others that are available. Known as NUTRIPLEX, Dr. Todd uses it as the basis for his nutritional treatment of cataracts. (See P. 201 for a listing of the ingredients in NUTRIPLEX.)

Dr. Lane's approach is to measure the status of the body's protective enzymes and biochemical indexes. He then suggests specific dietary changes based on these measurements. With this treatment, Dr. Lane can reverse cataract growth and restore vision to the level of health and degree of clarity it had one to two years prior to the start of treatment. For this reason, early detection and treatment is critical.

The cost of cataract prevention through nutritional supplements averages just $13.00 per month: That's 65 *years* of individual treatment for less than the cost of surgery! The health care implications are staggering.

(Another promising approach: The Chinese herb, Hachimijiogan, has been shown to increase the glutathione content of the lens. Hachimijiogan has been used for a long time in both China and Japan in the treatment of cataracts.)

Macular Degeneration

The macula is the part of the retina that is responsible for fine, detailed vision. A person with macular degeneration loses central vision and also has a poor recovery from exposure to bright lights. The loss of central vision is due either to a reduced blood supply to the central portion of the retina or to edema (a swelling and leakage of blood vessels in the retina).

Macular degeneration is the leading cause of severe vision loss in people aged 55 or older in the United States and Europe. At least 3 million Americans suffer irreversible vision loss from macular degeneration.

According to regular medicine, there is nothing that can be done to treat macular degeneration, although laser surgery is sometimes used to seal any leaking blood vessels. This surgery is successful only between 4 and 15% of the time (over a 5 year period). More importantly, it doesn't address the underlying conditions that might contribute to macular degeneration. (There is also a 50% possibility that a person's vision will be worse immediately after laser surgery.)

The primary underlying conditions in macular degeneration appear to be free radical damage and disrupted blood and oxygen supply to the macular region of the retina.

This would indicate that a nutritional approach that emphasized the anti-oxidant vitamins and minerals — vitamin C and E, zinc and selenium — could be helpful.

In fact, one study did show that 200 mg of zinc helped to improve acuity in people with macular degeneration. In another, people who have had higher levels of Vitamin E also had less vision loss that those with lower levels.

However, Dr. Todd believes that the underlying cause of macular degeneration (and also glaucoma) is an under-functioning thyroid. (There is a simple home test that anyone can perform to determine if they have an under-functioning thyroid. For complete details, send $1.00 to cover the cost of shipping and handling to: Cambridge Institute for Better Vision, 65 Wenham Road, Topsfield MA 01983.)

In addition to testing and balancing the functioning of the thyroid, Dr. Todd also suggests the following nutritional supplements on a daily basis:

Zinc Picolinate	**20 mg**
Selenium	**400 - 600 mcg**
Chromium	**200 mcg**
Vitamin A	**20,000 IU**
Natural Vitamin D *(not synthetic)*	**15,000 units**
Vitamin E	**400 - 1600 IU**
Vitamin C	**500 - 1000 mg**

Dr. Todd also recommends bioflavinoids (to reduce swelling of macular region), evening primrose (to re-establish integrity of vessel walls) and lecithin.

Although the anti-oxidant vitamins and minerals are important, the body needs zinc, copper, manganese and selenium to help control the free radicals. Yet, in his analysis of his patients, Dr. Todd has found that 60% are deficient in zinc, 15% in copper, 80 - 90% in manganese and that virtually everyone is deficient in selenium. These deficiencies greatly reduce the effectiveness of vitamins E and C and beta-carotene.

Dr. Todd will not treat anyone who won't stop smoking cigarettes, and he also recommends drinking only spring water, eliminating margarine and other hydrogenated fats and avoiding laser surgery, if at all possible. (He has found that people don't respond to nutritional approaches after having had laser surgery.)

When following his treatment approaches, 88% of Dr. Todd's patients improved vision significantly over a two-year period.

The herbs bilberry (Anthocyanosides) and Ginkgo biloba have been used extensively in Europe for many years to help eye conditions, including macular degeneration. Clinical studies have shown that both can inhibit progressive vision loss. According to some studies, these two herbs appear to work directly on the eye and are more potent than nutritional anti-oxidants.

Bilberry is also used for poor day and night vision, glaucoma and diabetic retinopathy. It has been shown to support the pigmented epithelium of the retina, reinforce the collagen structures and prevent free radical damage.

Gingko biloba increases the blood flow to the brain. European studies demonstrate impressive results in the treatment of macular degeneration and this herb has also been shown to prevent free radical damage to the retina and macula.

Glaucoma

Glaucoma is the leading cause of blindness in the United States, according to the American Academy of Ophthalmology. Approximately two million people are afflicted with glaucoma, with one out of every four cases going undetected.

Glaucoma goes undetected so often because it can develop without producing any noticeable symptoms.

Each eye is filled with a gelatinous fluid, called the vitreous humour (which has nothing to do with the tears on the outside the eye). This intraocular fluid is constantly being replenished and drained from the eye. The fluid is produced by the ciliary body (located behind the iris) which also controls the focusing of the lens. Glaucoma results from damage to the optic nerve.

One of the primary causes of optic nerve damage is the increase of pressure inside the eye. This increase destroys vision by putting pressure on the nerve and restricting blood supply and nutrient value to the optic nerve. The determining factor in glaucoma is the damage that results to the optic nerve, not necessarily the internal pressure of the eye. This damage leads to a loss of peripheral vision, permanent blind spots and, in the most severe cases, blindness.

Most often, the buildup of pressure occurs when the drainage system (called the trabecular network) for the fluid becomes partially blocked. Called **chronic** (open-angle) glaucoma, it is the most common form of glaucoma with over 90% of glaucoma patients having this type. There are usually no symptoms associated with the early stages of chronic glaucoma, so early detection — and prevention — is critical in preserving vision.

Acute (closed-angle) glaucoma occurs when the trabecular network becomes blocked suddenly and the intraocular pressure dramatically increases to dangerous levels. The pressure gets so high so fast that it must be treated as an emergency problem with surgery the only effective treatment.

Increase in pressure can also be caused by the increased production of fluid, though this is most rare.

Various activities affect eye pressure. For example, exercise lowers it, Eye Stretches (P. 84) can lower it, severe emotional stress can increase it, as can coffee, in people who already have glaucoma.

Certain vitamins can also affect pressure. Doctors at the University of Rome gave glaucoma patients megadoses of Vitamin C (1.5 grams for every 2.2 pounds of body weight), which resulted in a rapid and significant drop in intraocular pressure. In a trial of 26 people, a drop was noted in 17 who were given 20 mgs of rutin 3 times a day. Manganese (20 - 40 mgs/day) also can lower eye pressure.

For more than 10 years, it has been known that most patients with chronic glaucoma have a vitamin A deficiency. Many are also deficient in the enzyme, NAD, which also lowers eye pressure.

Nutritional treatment is helpful for sufferers of chronic glaucoma. According to Dr. Gary Price Todd, 25 - 40% of patients can be helped to some degree with an individualized nutritional program.

According to Dr. Todd, one critical key to nutritional treatment is increasing the body's levels of NAD. Normally, the body produces adequate levels of NAD, but if there is a deficiency in any of the critical trace minerals — such as copper, magnesium, manganese, selenium and zinc — NAD production levels are lowered. (Interestingly, Dr. Todd has examined over 2,000 patients and has found that more than 60% of them are deficient in one, or more, of these important trace minerals.) NAD levels can also be increased by taking Coenzyme Q-10.

Just as important to Dr. Todd as NAD levels is the functioning of the thyroid in glaucoma. Almost always, Dr. Todd finds that hypothyroidism — an under-functioning thyroid — is present in patients with chronic glaucoma.

Dr. Todd's comprehensive treatment for chronic glaucoma involves three steps:

1. Evaluate the functioning of the thyroid and treat if found to be under-functioning. (There is a simple home test that anyone can perform to determine if they have an under-functioning thyroid. For complete details, send $1.00 to cover the cost of shipping and handling to: Cambridge Institute for Better Vision, 65 Wenham Road, Topsfield MA 01983.)

2. Evaluate the level of trace minerals in the body and supplement as needed to bring all levels up to normal.

3. Suggest this daily nutritional program initially **in addition to NUTRIPLEX** (P. 201) and then re-evaluate after 2 - 3 months:

Coenzyme Q-10	**50 mg**
Vitamin A	**10,000 IU**
Vitamin D	**400 IU**
Vitamin C and Bioflavinoids	**1000 mg**
Biotin	**1000 mcg**
Magnesium	**100 mg**
Manganese chelate	**20 mg**
DMG (Dimethylglycine)	**250 mg**
Niacin	**80 - 200 mg**

One final point: Dr. Todd finds that people who do not respond to nutritional therapy may also have high levels of the toxic metal cadmium in their bodies. This heavy metal interferes with the body's absorption of vitamins and minerals, so Dr. Todd recommends that his glaucoma patients be tested for this as well.

Nutritional benefits are usually experienced in 2 to 3 months. Dr. Todd's patients have consistently been able to control glaucoma, restore some degree of lost vision, reduce the need for medication, and, in some cases, eliminate the need for it completely.

In Europe, the herbs bilberry and Gingko biloba have been tested and used for glaucoma treatment.

CHAPTER NINE

YOUR MIND AND YOUR EYES

To most completely understand how vision works, let's compare it to the process of producing a finished photograph. Because even after you've focused the lens and taken the picture, you still don't have a photograph until the film gets developed. This is done in the darkroom.

The darkroom in the brain

After an image is registered on the retina (film) it then has to be developed into a visual image (a photograph). This is done in the occipital region of the brain (the photographer's darkroom). (Fig. 6)

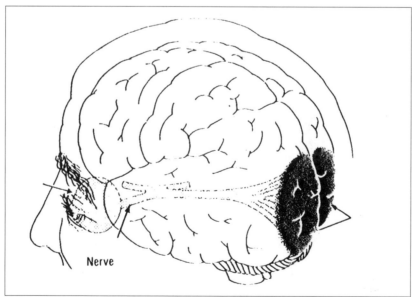

Nerve

Fig. 6   The 'darkroom' of the eye is the visual cortex - that part of the brain that produces visual images.

Vision — the formation of images of the physical world — does not occur until the brain receives impulses sent to it by the eyes. The darkroom of your visual system is a portion of the brain known as the visual cortex or the occipital lobe, which is located in the back of the head.

As everyone knows, the camera could take a perfect picture, but as a result of some error in processing the photograph could appear unclear or too dark or too light. Conversely, current space-age darkroom processing techniques can greatly enhance the quality of an under-developed picture, bringing out greater clarity, detail and brightness.

But the human darkroom — the visual processing center in the brain (particularly the occipital region) — can take an image that is blurred and make it clearer in the brain. This human darkroom is much more complex and intricate than any man-made darkroom.

How complex? As one example, the light that enters the eye hits the retina where the image registers upside-down. Fortunately the image is "righted" in the seeing centers of the brain, otherwise we would see the world upside-down. Vision, or the formation of images of the physical world, does not occur until the brain receives impulses sent to it by the eyes. This system is so complex that researchers still do not know exactly how the brain produces these visual images.

The photographer in each of us

The most striking omission of the eye/camera analogy is the complex role of the brain in the visual process.

In the case of the camera, it is the photographer who controls the camera — deciding what to shoot at, how much light to let in, what to focus on, for how long and from what angle.

In the case of the eye, each of us is our own photographer — and the choices we make about what we see and how we see are governed by the mysterious interplay between our physiological processes and our conscious and unconscious mental and emotional decisions.

Inner vision

Inner vision consists of two distinct aspects:

1. **Inner focus:** The attitudes and perspectives that form your view of yourself and the world.

2. **Visualization:** The ability to interpret or understand what is seen (i.e., to make meaning out of symbols) and the ability to produce images with the mind's eye. Visualization is strongly connected to memory.

Inner focus is best illustrated by the age-old example of two people looking at a glass of water. One sees it as half full, the other as half empty. The physical reality is the same, but the focus is different. Each person has a unique inner focus — the result of the interplay between memories, past experiences, attitudes and expectations.

The limiting and negative thoughts that we may have developed about our eyes can also affect how we see.

"I can't see" is probably the most common negative statement about vision. Just think how many times you've said that to yourself throughout the years — without even really thinking about it — *"I can't see," "I can't see without glasses," "I can't see that," "I can't see this,"* etc. etc.

Most people who have clear vision take it for granted. They don't necessarily think positively about their eyes. But if a person has a vision problem, they'll also start to develop a set of negative thoughts and attitudes about their eyes. In fact, cluster of negativity around vision and seeing often precedes — and sustains — a vision problem.

Of course, it would be foolish to tell ourselves we *can* see something when it isn't clear. But it's also very important to understand that there is a part of our body and mind that listens to — and responds to — what we tell ourselves.

Every time you put on glasses or contact lenses you are saying to yourself, *"I can't see without these."* When you say, *"I can't see,"* there's a part of you that believes it to be true. This, in turn, leads to your not even bothering to look at anything without them. The less you look, the less you see; the less you see, the less you look. The spiral continues. Downward.

Another learned bad habit is not bothering to look at the world without your glasses because you cannot see it clearly. To counter this, take the time to look into your "blur zone" — that part of your visual world that you are not yet seeing as clearly as you would like. Notice — and accept — what you are seeing. It may not be what you think you should be seeing, but relax, breathe easily and blink as you look. Notice what you can see and how you feel. The more you look, the more you see; the more you see, the more you look. The spiral continues. Upward.

The only time that it is truthful to say *"I can't see"* is when your eyes are completely closed. If your eyes are open **you are always seeing something**. If you focus on what you **can** see, you will want to look more often and more fully, which in turn will lead to seeing more. Relax and accept what you can see as you look around. And always acknowledge yourself for what you are seeing.

You can deliberately and consciously change your inner focus. *"My vision is always improving," "I'm looking for my vision to change," "My vision is becoming clearer and clearer every day"* and *"I want to see more"* are all just as "true" in describing your current situation, but they also reinforce the possibility of change.

(To fully put the power of Vision Affirmations to work for you, see Pp. 167 - 169) for complete instructions.)

Many scientists and medical professionals already understand and appreciate that the condition of the body is affected by the content of the thoughts and the nature of the feelings. And, if you start to change these mental and emotional patterns for yourself, the body — and the eyes — responds.

Unfortunately, it's not as simple as saying *"I want to see"* once and then having your vision become perfectly clear. That is an important first step but most often the habit patterns that you want to change go deeper. It is what we hold to be true subconsciously and emotionally that has the most profound effect on how we see. Consistent efforts at releasing negative thoughts and emotional barriers and practicing positive visualization can change the deeper subconscious patterns. (See the next chapter, **Your Emotions and Your Eyes**.)

Visualization, perhaps the highest level of visual skill, is an act of creation and can be an awesome tool if used, directed and finely tuned.

For example, without visualization you would be unable to read. You might be able to see the letters "c", "a" and "t", which make up the word "cat," but only when you produce the image of a cat in your brain/mind do those letters take on any meaning.

What you visualize or imagine directly influences your physical body. In fact, your body cannot tell the difference between what the imagination tells it and what is "real."

Consider the physical and emotional reactions to a nightmare. Your palms sweat, your heart pounds and you feel afraid. That's the same reaction you'd have if you "really" saw what you had just dreamed.

Vision research indicates that the focusing mechanism of the eye physically responds to what the imagination is focusing on. If the mind imagines looking at a distant mountain, the eye changes its focus as if it were actually looking at a distant mountain.

A classic psychological study demonstrates the beneficial effects of visualization. In it a group of basketball players were tested for free throw accuracy before and after a 20-day period. The first group practiced free throws 20 minutes a day for 20 days, the second did not practice at all and the third spent 20 minutes a day "visualizing" themselves practicing.

The result? The group that actually practiced and the group that visualized practicing improved virtually to the same degree.

The **Mind's Eye Visualization** (P.90) trains you to use the incredible power of visualization to help improve your vision. During the visualization, you are asked to close your eyes in your imagination, feel them relaxing and then to re-open your eyes again in your imagination.

One man wrote The Cambridge Institute describing his experience the first time that he did the **Mind's Eye Visualization**. He misunderstood the instructions as he was listening to the visualization on audiotape and in error he actually opened his eyes, instead of just *imagining* that he was opening them while doing the visualization.

When he mistakenly opened his eyes, his vision was perfectly clear! This spell of clear vision lasted for only a few minutes, but it convinced him that he did in fact have the ability to see clearly.

(This audiotape and others are available to you. See Pp. 199 - 202 for more information.)

The brain/mind and the eyes are designed to function together. When the mind is preoccupied, daydreaming or uninvolved the eyes are caught between the imagination and physical reality and they function less effectively. Prolonged daydreaming — visualizing or imagining one thing while your eyes are seeing something else — creates visual and mental strain.

If you catch yourself daydreaming, bored or preoccupied, stop, take a deep breath, and re-focus physically and mentally on what you are seeing. Become more present, more aware and more involved. Or, if you want to continue daydreaming, close your eyes.

That's the difference between seeing and looking. Your eyes may be seeing, but you may not be looking. The difference between seeing and looking is involvement, an essential ingredient of visual clarity.

With the proper use of your inner vision and the development of your ability to visualize you can considerably shorten the time it takes to learn to develop **Better Vision**.

CHAPTER TEN

YOUR EMOTIONS AND YOUR EYES

Our eyes are sensitive emotional receptors through which we relate to other human beings. We express our feelings through our eyes. We can often tell what someone else is thinking by the "look" in his/her eyes. And, in many ways, how we feel tempers how and what we see.

Statements such as *"What you don't see won't hurt you," "Blind with rage,"* or *"I wish that problem would disappear,"* address emotional seeing; so does not looking at or forgetting to see certain part of ourselves — both positive and negative.

The eyes have been called "the windows of the soul." As we open our eyes and honestly look at ourselves and others, we can experience a deeper sense of connectedness to and understanding of ourselves and others.

The Transitional Period

The underlying causes of not seeing clearly can often rest in the emotional and mental levels of vision. Changes in eyesight can be preceded by major changes in feelings, attitudes or perspective.

To see how this works, divide your life into three periods: The time when you had clear vision, the time that you have spent with poor vision (needing glasses or contacts) and the transition time between these two.

Glasses and contacts represent an attempt to deal with the symptoms — not the causes — of not seeing clearly. Furthermore, the entire period of time (Period C) spent needing glasses does not address any of the initial reasons that led to needing them in the first place.

Natural clear vision	The Transitional Period	Needing to use glasses
BIRTH _____	_____	_____CURRENT AGE
Period A	**Period B**	**Period C**

Vision is a learned process that develops in a child much the same as learning to walk. Whether it is consciously remembered or not, almost everyone has experienced a period of time (Period A) with natural clear vision. (Remember, poor vision is not inherited!)

To understand the inner causes of unclear vision it is necessary to look at the **Transitional Period** (Period B) — the time (usually a year though it could be longer) between seeing clearly with natural eyes to first noticing a limitation in physical vision. (Some people do not get glasses or contacts as soon as there is a visual limitation, so it is important to note that the **Transitional Period** is the year or so that precedes the visual limitation, not necessarily the time that you first got glasses.)

The lessening of physical clarity can represent changes in our own emotional, subconscious and psychological responses to ourselves — or to the world around us — that become ingrained during this **Transitional Period**.

Most people can identify a transition in at least one of three major areas in the period before they first needed glasses.

    1. Personal: Changes in self image usually (but not always) accompanied by physical changes during adolescence (reaching puberty) or with middle age (aging). Or changes in the fundamental ways in which other people or life are perceived.

    2. Emotional: Changes in significant relationships. (Parents divorce, another child is born or a loved one dies.)

3. Situational: Changes in the environment. (Moving to another town and having to make new friends or staying in the same town but switching careers, homes or schools.)

Whatever the specific external changes may have been, it is the inner changes — of feelings, attitudes or perspective — that are most important and significant. The emotional and subconscious statement, *"I don't want to see this part of myself or this problem,"* can affect the visual system. Exactly how is not yet clear, but the effect is real.

During this **Transitional Period** a person usually doesn't want to admit to what is being seen, sensed or perhaps even feared. The message, *"I don't want to see what is going on,"* is sent to the subconscious mind. Delivered with emotion, this message becomes a command to the mind to develop a more limited pattern of seeing. The visual system responds accordingly. Not wanting to be seen or hiding from others out of fear or shame also contributes to the closing and limiting of the visual system.

Impact of the Transitional Period

Addressing the inner decisions made during the **Transitional Period** can have a profound — and sometimes immediate — effect on one's physical eyesight.

For example, one middle-aged stockbroker who had been unable to read anything without his glasses looked back at his **Transitional Period** — a time when he was losing money in the stock market. He recalled that he had finally reached the point where he was afraid to look at the stock tables for *"fear of seeing"* how much he had lost that day. The tables had become the *"proof"* to him that he was a failure and that was what he didn't want to see.

While using **The Memory Visualization** (Pp. 97 - 101) and related techniques he realized that he had formed an image of himself as being *"a failure."* When he was able to let go of that false image he recognized that his sense of himself went deeper than the ups and downs of the stock market. He saw himself as more than his temporary successes or failures. His vision returned to normal and he began to read and work without glasses for the first time in five years.

Another example is that of a woman who attended The Cambridge Institute's EYECLASSES Vision Seminar. For two years prior to the seminar she had been involved in vision training with a leading eye specialist.

During this two year period her distance acuity had improved from 20/400 to 20/200. But in the Seminar she did something that she had never done before — she healed some of the emotional memories that were locked in her subconscious since her **Transitional Period**.

Three days after the seminar she went back to her doctor and her visual acuity had improved from 20/200 to 20/80 — a greater improvement in 2 days than she had achieved in 2 years! Needless to say, both she and her doctor were quite surprised and thrilled.

Developing the emotional willingness to see can have a definite impact on vision.

Now if you can go further back in time than the **Transitional Period**, that is the time of natural, clear vision (Part A). The ability to see clearly may still be inside of us and our subconscious brain may "remember" how to see clearly. Even if that memory may be buried underneath negative thinking and emotional stress, it's there waiting to re-emerge.

Unresolved emotional issues, particularly those involving loss, fear and misunderstanding, coupled with the attendant forgetting of one's deeper positive qualities — such as acceptance, compassion and forgiveness — are also key elements of the **Transitional Period**.

All of us have been in situations where we see things we don't like or that have hurt us in some way. One response is to pull back or push away; to shut down our awareness. There's a part of ourselves that imagines, *"If I pretend not to see it, it will disappear."* Pretending not to see or not to know is one strategy to deal with oneself, one's feelings or one's life situation. It may be a useful protection at certain times, but one of its by-products is the way it can affect eyesight, both immediately and over the long run.

Recovering from early emotional decisions and healing painful memories greatly accelerates vision improvement and also leads to a greater sense of inner peace and understanding, a clearer self image, and a healthier attitude and perspective.

Some people stop themselves from gaining greater emotional clarity by saying they can't remember anything "back then." That's understandable, because there is a link between memory, vision and imagination. But when you start to improve your vision, your memory of significant events becomes clearer as well.

Once you start exploring the connection between your emotions, your memories and your vision, you will be surprised at what — and how much — you see.

PART 2

GETTING READY

CHAPTER ELEVEN

DECIDING HOW TO USE
YOUR GLASSES AND CONTACTS

NOTE: NEVER DRIVE WITHOUT YOUR GLASSES OR CONTACTS UNLESS YOU CAN PASS YOUR STATE DRIVER'S LICENSE TEST WITHOUT THEM.

All of the information in this section applies equally to the use of contacts.

Quantifiable vision improvement will be difficult to achieve unless you change the way you are presently using your glasses or contacts. What kind of glasses or contacts you use and how you use them are key factors that will increase — or hinder — the speed of your improvement.

Which glasses to use

Some people can improve their vision by using their current glasses less and less. Others need to take the intermediate step of using an under-corrected — or weaker — prescription.

Here's how to decide which is the best way for you to proceed:

If your current prescription is very strong, taking off your glasses altogether might actually hinder improvement because the initial strain and stress that caused the need for glasses is still present. Straining or "trying to see" to make a blurry world seem clearer also prevents improvement.

If you are nearsighted and need to use glasses for more than 2 - 4 hours a day, then you should get an under-corrected prescription. **If you are farsighted** and absolutely cannot read or do other close work without glasses, then you, too, should get an under-corrected prescription, regardless of how few hours a day you use glasses.

The under-corrected prescription will give you enough clarity for most activities (including driving), but leave "room" for your own natural vision to improve. For nearsighted people, this under-corrected prescription will usually give a distance acuity of 20/40. If you are farsighted or presbyopic, have your reading glasses changed to the near-range equivalent of 20/40.

An alternative to getting a weaker prescription may be to use an older pair of glasses. Though usually viable, this alternative might not always be appropriate. For instance, if the older glasses had a correction for an astigmatism that has since changed, it would be wiser to first have a new examination with an optometrist.

As your natural vision improves, what was once an under-corrected prescription will eventually become too strong and you will require still another weaker prescription. This gradual "weaning" from glasses has two distinct advantages:

1. You can go about your daily activities without difficulty

2. The weaker prescription will reduce any unconscious straining that you might be doing.

Not every optometrist will comply with your request for an under-corrected prescription, though it might be easier than you think to find one who will. Within the field of optometry there is a specially trained group of doctors who practice vision training. These doctors, known as behavioral optometrists, will usually cooperate with the request for an under-correction. (See the next chapter, **Visiting The Eye Doctor**.)

How to use your glasses

Always look for ways to reduce the amount of time you use your glasses, whether they are under-corrected or not.

It is important to remember not to strain or squint when you are without glasses. Instead, cultivate the attitude of visual acceptance. Notice what you can see and what you are seeing, without comparing it to what you think you should see.

If you don't get a weaker prescription then it's imperative to go without glasses a majority of the time if you want to significantly improve your vision.

There are many adjustments you can make to increase your time without glasses. For instance, mornings, consciously delay the time when you first put on your glasses. On the telephone, take off your glasses. On auto trips, don't use your glasses unless you're at the wheel yourself. Or, at the movies, sit closer. If you're farsighted, light the room better when reading, or read in natural light. Keep looking for situations in which you can use your natural vision.

If you use contacts it is much harder to practice this "on again, off again" approach. We strongly recommend that you either switch to glasses or that you get an under-corrected prescription for your contact lenses.

In addition, it is important to spend at least 20 - 30 minutes a day outside without using any glasses or contacts at all. This allows the full spectrum of sunlight to enter your body through the eyes, which is beneficial to your eyes as well as to your overall health and well-being. Protection from over-exposure to UV light may be necessary if you spend a lot of time outdoors, but a healthy, regular dose of natural, unfiltered sunlight is vital to your health and your eyesight.

CHAPTER TWELVE

VISITING THE EYE DOCTOR

Picture a visit to the optometrist or ophthalmologist and what do you think of? An eye chart on the wall on one side of the examining room and you in a chair on the opposite side trying to read the tiny letters on the bottom line, first with one eye then with the other.

And, if you can read the bottom line, your vision is perfect. If you can't, you need glasses. Right?

Not necessarily!

Good vision is much more than just 20/20.

Even if you have 20/20 (with or without correction), there could still exist other deficiencies in the visual system that would go undetected during a simple test for visual acuity. And if these deficiencies continue to go unnoticed, they could eventually lead to problems with acuity. So a person could end up needing glasses (or stronger glasses) when the real causes of the problem are going uncorrected.

Problems in these other areas might cause some of the following symptoms: double vision, headaches, tiredness, poor depth perception, difficulty concentrating while reading, eyestrain, burning, stinging, dry eyes, and more.

Balanced visual functioning requires that the eyes move easily from point to point and work together as a team, that the brain can effectively use peripheral vision and that the brain can easily process visual information.

Using glasses that were prescribed after only a test for distance or near-point acuity could very likely lead to further visual stress. If there are other undetected visual problems that remain unaddressed, this could lead to prescriptions that get stronger and stronger, deteriorating vision and a general feeling of discomfort and fatigue. All of which could set the stage for even more serious eye problems to develop.

That's why it is so important to get a complete and thorough examination from a doctor who understands the interconnectedness of all aspects of vision.

Here is a list of the vision checks and tests that a behavioral optometrist will most likely perform during the first visit:

- Measure distance vision with an eye chart.
- Determine how your eyes function at close range.
- Measure the teamwork between your eyes and your brain.
- See how smoothly your eyes move from point to point.
- See how smoothly and easily your eyes follow a moving target.
- See how easily each eye can shift focus from near to far.
- Screen for medical conditions like glaucoma and cataracts.

Finding The Right Optometrist

How can you find an optometrist that can give you a complete and thorough examination?

First of all, look for a behavioral optometrist.

A behavioral optometrist is a doctor who believes that how you see is the result of how you have learned to use your eyes and that visual skills — including how clearly you can see — can be enhanced through exercise, relaxation and training. He/she has received specialized training, can give you a comprehensive examination, and can perform all the tests listed above.

Of course, a behavioral optometrist, like a regular optometrist, can prescribe glasses and contacts. But a behavioral optometrist would be more likely to comply with your request for an under-corrected prescription. In addition, a behavioral optometrist can provide a program of training that improves overall visual functioning.

The Cambridge Institute maintains a nationwide **Select Referral List** of behaviorally oriented optometrists. For help in finding one in your area, contact:

Cambridge Institute for Better Vision

65 Wenham Road

Topsfield MA 01983

(508) 887-3883

Other organizations that may be helpful to you in your search are:

College of Optometrists in Vision Development	**Optometric Extension Program Foundation**
P.O. Box 285	2912 S. Daimler Street
Chula Vista, CA 92012	Santa Ana, CA 92705
(619) 425-6191	(714) 250-8070

However you find a behavioral optometrist, the most important element is to find one who not only agrees with the principles in this book, but also uses them in some way in his or her practice.

When you have the name of someone, it is perfectly reasonable to phone the doctor and ask whether he or she does the complete series of tests described. It is also useful to inquire whether vision therapy is available in the office; the fact it is indicates that the doctor most likely is behaviorally oriented. It is also permissible to ask if the doctor would be willing, after an examination, to prescribe an under-corrected prescription.

If you want an under-corrected prescription, even if you cannot locate a behavioral optometrist, it's possible that a regular optometrist would be willing to comply with your request after an examination. It is your right as a patient to ask!

If the doctor that you visit has any questions, have them call the Cambridge Institute directly (508-887-3883). We should be able to give them the information that they need to help you. This way, you are not putting yourself in the position of having to explain something to someone else that you might not yet completely understand yourself.

CHAPTER THIRTEEN

SETTING UP YOUR PRACTICE AREA

NOTE: ALL PRACTICE SESSIONS ARE TO BE COMPLETED WITHOUT GLASSES OR CONTACT LENSES.

Choose a place to practice where you feel comfortable and won't be disturbed. It would be best if your practice area had natural light, but sufficient artificial light is fine. You'll need to attach your Fusion String to the wall at eye level and be able to sit or stand 6 - 8 feet away. (See Pp. 64 - 68, Fusion String Technique, for more details.)

Also, attach the Vision Chart that you will be using to the wall so that the center of the chart is at eye level. Make sure there is no glare on the chart. You will need a space large enough to stand or sit the appropriate distance from the chart. (See P. 79, **Which Vision Chart to Use**, for more details.) You will also need enough room (approximately 3 feet square) to stand and Swing (P. 70).

The importance of practice

The key to improving your vision successfully is regular and consistent practice. Regular sessions serve two purposes.

1. They develop the skills necessary for clear vision and reduce the amount of visual stress accumulated each day

2. They build a "consciousness of seeing" by nurturing and developing positive visual attitudes and habits.

Getting started may be the toughest part, but once you have your routine in place you'll look forward to each session. The momentum of these practice sessions builds.

Choosing a practice time

Any practice time works!

Make your vision important enough to have a place in your everyday life. If your session becomes something to fit in when you have the time, you might never practice.

Some people find it best to get the practice session out of the way before the regular demands of the day take up their time. Others find that after a busy day, practice is relaxing, beneficial and often revitalizing. Still others are tired after work and can't concentrate as well at the end of the day as they can at the beginning.

It is more productive to practice when you are fresh, but bear in mind that practicing tired is infinitely better than not practicing at all. Pick the time that you can be as fully involved as possible — free of distractions and with your privacy protected — and set a regular time to do your daily practice.

Committing time to practice on a regular basis is actively demonstrating to yourself your intention to change the way you see. It's never true that you can't find the time for the daily session. But it may be true that you won't/don't make the time. Don't kid yourself about the choice.

The only thing that keeps people from improving their vision is their lack of desire, motivation and discipline. Your willingness to do the work required, your belief in yourself while doing it, and your perseverance throughout will be major factors in successfully achieving your vision goals.

The Program for Better Vision works. Engage **The Program** with "the eyes of a child" — with a freshness and a sense of excitement — and it will work for you.

PART 3

THE FIRST STAGE 8-WEEK SCHEDULE

CHAPTER FOURTEEN

THE SIX VISION SESSIONS

THE FIRST STAGE is an 8-week schedule that guides you towards **Better Vision**. You practice only one Vision Session each day, according to the schedule.

There are six different Vision Sessions:

Vision Session 1: **Fusion String Technique** (Pp. 64 - 68)
Vision Session 2: **Self-Massage Techniques** (Pp. 69 - 78)
Vision Session 3: **Vision Chart Techniques** (Pp. 79 - 89)
Vision Session 4: **Mind's Eye Visualization** (Pp. 90 - 92)
Vision Session 5: **Spectrum Visualization** (Pp. 93 - 96)
Vision Session 6: **Memory Visualization** (Pp. 97 - 101)

The Self-Massage Techniques and Vision Chart Techniques each contain a series of individual exercises. The other four Vision Sessions contain only one visualization or technique.

The instructions for the Vision Sessions are in the next section. **THE FIRST STAGE** 8-week daily schedule follows that.

The six Vision Sessions work with a variety of improvement techniques for the physical, mental and emotional levels of your vision.

Once you become familiar with the instructions, each Vision Session should take between 15 and 25 minutes to complete.

General tips

Here are some tips to keep in mind when you are practicing the Vision Sessions:

1. To achieve the maximum benefit, practice with awareness and relaxed concentration. The techniques will help you release visual stress and change the visual habits that cause poor vision. Their effectiveness will probably be dramatically reduced if you practice in a mechanical fashion.

2. Practice **without** your glasses or contact lenses.

3. Before you begin make sure that you read the section on Correct Posture (Pp. 21 - 23). Most of the techniques can be practiced either in a sitting or standing position.

4. Do not strain or "try to see." This attitude of effort will only impede your progress. Relax as you use your eyes to see.

5. The time and repetitions allocated for each exercise are guidelines only. They suggest the general pace at which to do the exercise; feel free to spend more time on any exercise that you feel is particularly helpful. Don't rush.

Keep these tips in mind when practicing the visualizations:

1. After you make sure that you won't be disturbed, sit in a comfortable position with your arms and legs uncrossed. Loosen any tight clothing, close your eyes, take a few deep breaths and relax.

2. Don't be concerned if at first your mind drifts or wanders or your concentration fades. Your concentration will improve as you continue doing these visualizations. Developing visual skills (i.e. your imagination) takes practice and patience.

3. It is helpful to play relaxing background music during the visualization.

4. It is common to fall asleep during part or all of these visualizations. This is a normal sign of deep relaxation. As you grow accustomed to the relaxed state you will find it easier to remain awake. Do not lie down while doing the visualizations if you have a tendency to fall asleep. If you fall asleep too often while seated, experiment by doing the visualizations while standing.

5. It is most effective to have someone guide you through the visualizations. You can have a partner do that or you can record your voice on audiotape and listen to the visualization that way. Or, you can receive the visualizations already recorded on audiotape (with pleasing background music) from The Cambridge Institute for Better Vision (P. 199).

INSTRUCTIONS FOR THE SIX VISION SESSIONS

Vision Session One:

FUSION STRING TECHNIQUE

Vision Session One, **Fusion String Technique**, contains one exercise (using the Fusion String).

Purpose

1. To develop binocularity — the ability of the mind and eyes to work together.

2. To develop convergence — the ability of both eyes to look at the same point .

3. To develop accommodation — the ability to change focus from one point to another.

REPETITIONS   10 times with both eyes (up and down the Fusion String) then 5 more times (with each eye)

TIME 20 minutes

MATERIALS One Fusion String

You can make your own string by stringing 10 beads on a seven-foot long string. The beads should be six inches apart. (Or you can get a Fusion String from the Cambridge Institute, 65 Wenham Road, Topsfield, MA 01983. Include $3.00 for handling.)

SET UP

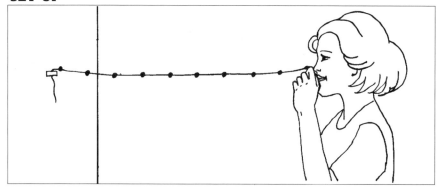

Fig. 7 Attach one end of the Fusion String to the wall slightly below eye level.

1. Attach one end of the Fusion String to the wall with a piece of tape or a push pin at a height slightly lower than eye level. Good illumination is critical. Wrap the free end of the Fusion String around your index finger and hold the string up to the tip of your nose. The string should make a straight but slightly downward line from

your nose to the wall. Do not lean forward or tilt backwards to make the string straight. Instead, step a little closer to, or farther away from, the wall. (Fig. 7)

Instructions

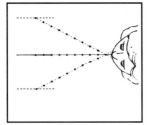

Fig. 8A When focused on your nose, you'll see two images of the String meeting in a V at your nose.

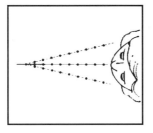

Fig. 8B When focused on the wall, you'll see two images of the String meeting at the wall in a V.

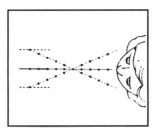

Fig. 8C When you focus on a particular bead, you'll see two images of the String crossing to form an X, with that bead the center of the X.

1. First, look at your nose and see the illusion of two strings meeting in a "V" at your nose. Blink and breathe. Use your peripheral vision. (Fig. 8A)

2. Now, shift your gaze to the wall where the string attaches. This time, see the illusion of two strings meeting in a "V" at the wall. (Fig. 8B)

3. Next, shift your vision to bead #5 and see the illusion of two strings crossing in an "X" over bead #5, with the center of the "X" directly on bead #5. (Fig. 8C)

4. Now slide your gaze to bead #1 (closest to nose) and focus on it. The illusion of the two strings meeting in an "X" is now there, with the center of the "X" on bead #1.

Continue sliding your gaze down the string — to bead #2, then #3, etc., all the way to bead #10 (closest to wall), focusing on each bead and at each bead seeing the illusion of the two strings meeting in an "X", with the center of the "X" directly on the bead at which you are looking.

After you finish bead #10, look at the wall and see the illusion of two strings meeting in a "V" at the wall.

5. Now, reverse direction, starting at bead #10, to bead #9, then #8, etc., all the way to bead #1 (closest to nose). After you finish bead #1, look at your nose and again see the illusion of two strings meeting there in a "V".

6. Close your eyes and let your hand drop from your nose. Turn your head slowly from side to side to relax your neck, shoulders and face. Turn your head 6 times.

REPEAT steps 4 - 6 eight more times.

7. Then cover your right eye with your hand (keeping the covered eye open) and repeat steps 4 - 6 four times. (See Palming, P. 78)

8. Then cover your left eye with your hand (keeping the covered eye open) and repeat steps 4 - 6 four more times.

What to watch for

1. Sometimes instead of seeing the "X" crossover at the bead people:

- See only one string instead of two;

- See two strings crossing in an "X", but the string crosses farther away from the bead;

- See two strings crossing in an "X", but the string crosses in front of the bead;

- See two strings crossing at some point and continuing in one string, so a "Y" is seen rather than an "X";

- See two strings that do not cross at all (which represents the absence of convergence abilities);

- See one string more solidly (darker or clearer) than the other. (To learn which eye is doing the seeing, alternately close each eye and notice which string disappears.)

2. Being unable to move the "X" farther away from or closer to a specific point is a sign that your convergence ability is stuck. (The former is usually associated with nearsightedness, the latter with farsightedness and middle-age sight.)

3. At first, improvement may not come in the form of clarity but in your being able to see and move the "X" within larger and larger areas on the string.

4. Holding your breath is feedback that you are straining or "trying to see," which always produces unclear vision. Remember to blink regularly, breathe fully and keep your body relaxed.

5. Forcing yourself to see almost always will lead to frustration and/or discouragement. Accept your vision. Notice what you can see. Acknowledge yourself for it. Be patient. Relax.

6. Be aware of objects in your peripheral vision.

Variations:

1. To help nearsightedness, go out the String only: Start with your focus on bead #1 and go out the string bead by bead. When you reach the wall, start again at bead #1. Continue in this manner, going out the string bead by bead, then re-starting at #1.

2. To help farsightedness, come in the String only: Start with your focus on bead #10 and come in the string bead by bead. When you reach bead #1, start again at bead #10. Continue in this manner, coming in the string bead by bead, then re-starting at #10.

3. To help astigmatism, set yourself up in the regular position, hold the string stationary and turn your head part way to the left. Practice by moving up and down the string as you would normally. Then turn your head part way to the right and practice normally. Continue practicing normally with your head tilted up slightly and then tilted down slightly.

Notes

1. As you move your eyes up and down the Fusion String, slide your gaze (instead of jumping) from bead to bead and pay the most attention to the crossover areas — places where the "X" stops following your mind's commands.

For example, if you're able to make the "X" cross at beads #1, #2, #3 and #4, but when you look at bead #5 the "X" seems to be stuck at bead #4, then slide your gaze back and forth over the crossover point between beads #4 and #5. Always work toward sliding the "X" further away from you or closer to you, whichever the direction of your improvement.

2. Issue verbal commands (out loud or silently) to your eyes when they do not place the "X" where you want it. Commands such as *"Eyes, focus where I tell you," "Eyes, look at where my mind wants you to,"* and *"See the 'X',"* are effective and will accelerate your progress.

3. If there is a bead that you cannot see, look at where you imagine that bead to be. In fact, if you carefully look at that area, you may see a glint of light reflecting off the bead or a hazy color of the bead. Do not force yourself to see more; instead, **always notice what you are seeing**. The more that you look, the more you will see. Remember, breathe regularly and concentrate on relaxing your shoulders, the back of your neck and the back of your head. Be patient with yourself.

4. With only one eye open, you'll see only one string. Moving each eye up and down the string will help you develop better accommodation and sharpen visual acuity.

5. When you palm over one eye, cup your palm over your eye with your free hand making sure your palm and eye/eyelid do not touch. Keep your palmed eye open.

6. If your hand gets tired, switch the hand that's holding the Fusion String to your nose. When you close your eyes, rest the String on your lap.

7. When turning your head from side to side, relax your shoulders and neck and breathe regularly and easily. Turn your head as far as you can with ease — do not strain.

8. When standing, make sure that your weight is equally distributed on both feet.

Vision Session Two:

SELF MASSAGE TECHNIQUES

Vision Session Two, **Self Massage Techniques**, is a series of eight exercises:

        1. Swinging

        2. Head Rolls

        3. Finger Tapping

        4. Five-Finger Eye Massage

        5. Three-Finger Eye Massage

        6. Energy Transfer Point Massage

        7. Occipital Point Massage

        8. Palming

1. Swinging

Purpose

1. To develop and regain the natural, easy movement of your eyes.

2. To relax your eyes and your upper body.

REPETITIONS 100

TIME 4 - 5 minutes

Instructions

1. With your knees relaxed and slightly bent, stand with your legs a little wider than your shoulder width apart.

2. Begin swinging your body from side to side, keeping your spine straight. Swing, don't sway. (Fig. 9)

The concept is to swing the upper body — torso, chest and head — as a unit around the axis of the spine, letting your head follow the movement of your body. Think of your body as moving like a flag with your spine the flagpole — so that as you rotate your spine remains in a straight line.

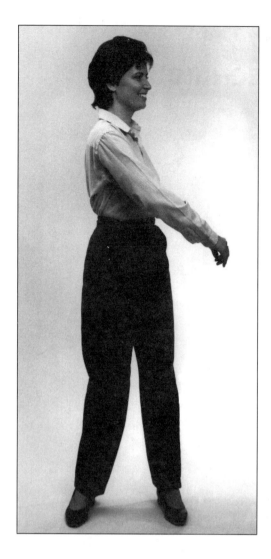

Fig. 9   SWINGING relaxes your eyes and body and helps re-develop the easy, natural movement of your eyes.

3. Let your eyes move freely and easily, following a line of sight parallel to the floor. Avoid looking down or tilting your head.

4. Do not "try to see" anything. Notice the motion, but let the world go by.

5. Relax your neck, shoulders, mid-back and stomach. Let your elbows bend naturally as you swing.

6. Swing at a relaxed speed.

7. Breathe regularly and easily and blink lightly and often in a relaxed manner.

What to watch for

1. A sign that you are letting go and not "trying to see" occurs when you notice the room spinning in the opposite direction than you are swinging. Prior to this, it may seem as if the room is not moving at all or that your focus is jumping from point to point "trying to hold onto" your visual world.

2. If you experience loss of balance, dizziness or nausea as you swing, redirect your awareness to 1) breathing regularly and deeply, 2) bending your knees and feeling your feet "grounded" (on the floor), and 3) seeing the room spinning in the opposite direction.

If the discomfort is too much to breathe through, stop, take a few deep breaths, re-orient yourself and — when it feels comfortable — start again.

2. Head Rolls

Purpose

To relax your neck, head and face muscles and reduce shoulder tension.

REPETITIONS 6 times (in each direction)
TIME 2 minutes

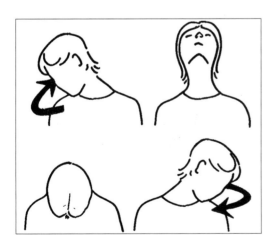

Fig. 10 HEAD ROLLS help to relax your neck and shoulders - two areas that can block clear vision. Remember to gently rotate your head and not to force any movements.

Instructions

1. Take a deep breath and, on the exhale, slowly drop your chin to your chest.

2. Inhale again deeply and as you do slowly roll your head to one side, around and up. Exhale freely as you roll your head around to the other side and down to your chest again. (Fig. 10)

3. Repeat 5 more times.

4. Reverse direction and repeat 6 more times.

What to watch for

1. Keep your shoulders still and relaxed and move only your head and neck.

2. Stiffness during certain movements of your head. Be gentle with yourself. Don't force any movements. How large the rolls are is not as important as doing them slowly and in a relaxed, easy manner.

3. Finger Tapping

Purpose

To stimulate the visual centers of your brain and develop the ability to focus clearly.

REPETITIONS 200
TIME 1 minute

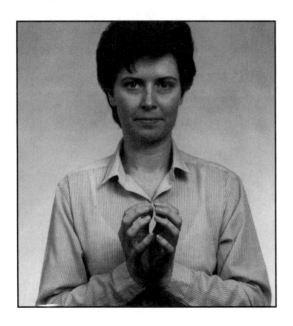

Fig. 11 FINGER TAPPING stimulates the nerve endings in the fingertips and the visual pathways in the brain.

Instructions

1. Loosely place the bottom of your palms together and, with your wrists relaxed, tap your finger*tips* together rapidly. (Fig. 11)

2. Breathe easily and keep your arms and elbows relaxed.

What to watch for

1. Tingling or tenderness in your fingertips. (This is a completely natural sensation.)

2. Sensations in other areas of your body, particularly the stomach region. These will disappear as body tension releases.

4. Five-Finger Eye Massage

Purpose

To stimulate the muscles that control the focusing mechanisms and lenses of your eyes.

REPETITIONS 1 time
TIME 1 - $1\frac{1}{2}$ minutes

Instructions

NOTE: THERE IS NO NEED TO WORRY OR FEAR; IT IS SAFE TO DO THIS MASSAGE TECHNIQUE.

1. Place the five fingertips of each hand together — as if you were cupping your fingers around a marble — and place them on your closed eyes. (Fig. 12)

2. Making very light contact between your eyes and your fingertips, massage both (closed) eyes by vibrating your fingertips lightly and quickly from side to side.

3. When you stop — and before you open your eyes — take a deep breath, exhale and, in a quick motion, fling your fingers away from your body as if you were throwing the tension away through your fingertips. Open your eyes.

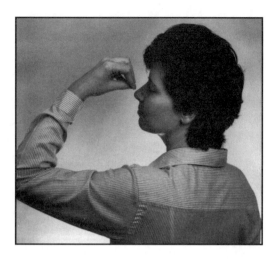

Fig. 12 FIVE-FINGER EYE MASSAGE is a safe way to massage the eyes, loosening tension and stimulating the visual system.

What to watch for

1. Using light pressure on your eyes. (Be sensitive and gentle when touching your eyes.)

2. Your eyes beginning to feel softer as you continue massaging them on a regular basis.

5. Three-Finger Eye Massage

Purpose

To stimulate the muscles that control the focusing mechanisms and lenses of your eyes.

REPETITIONS 5 times
TIME 1 minute

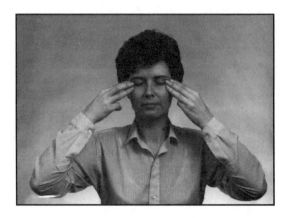

Fig. 13 THREE-FINGER EYE MASSAGE stimulates the focusing system in your eyes.

Instructions

1. Place the tips of each of your middle fingers on the bony outer corners of your eye sockets.

2. Close your eyes and gently hook both middle fingertips around and slightly inside these corners. Rest your index fingers on your temples, the other fingers on your cheeks and your thumbs behind your ears. Don't touch your eyes, just the inside surfaces of the outer corners of the sockets. (Fig. 13)

3. For a count of five, inhale and apply pressure in an outward direction on both sides simultaneously (as if trying to widen your head). Then, relax the pressure and exhale for a count of five.

4. Repeat four more times.

5. When you're done, fling your fingers away from your body — as if you are throwing the tension out of your body through your fingertips.

What to watch for
Applying firm (not hard) pressure.

6. Energy Transfer Point Massage

Purpose
1. To massage the Energy Transfer Points (ETPs) that channel the body's energy to your head, neck and eyes.
2. To increase the oxygen supply to your visual system.
3. To relax and release physical tension that affects your vision.

REPETITIONS 1 time (each side)
TIME 2 minutes (1 minute each side)

Instructions

1. Locate the ETP by bringing your left hand to your right shoulder near the base of your neck. Press deeply along the top ridge of your shoulder muscle until you find a

point that is tender, more sensitive or more stiff than the surrounding areas. That point may be pea-sized or much larger. (Fig. 14)

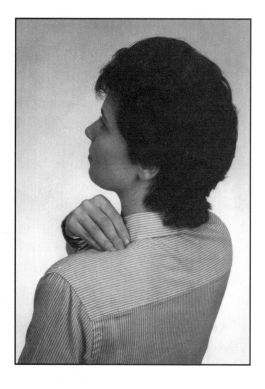

Fig. 14 ENERGY TRANSFER POINT MASSAGE releases shoulder and neck tension that can block energy flow to the eyes and brain.

2. Apply deep (but not painful) vibrating pressure to the ETP for approximately 1 minute. Go as deeply as is comfortable for you.

3. Breathe deeply and rhythmically, relaxing your neck, shoulder, arm and free hand.

4. Reverse and repeat.

What to watch for

1. Being gentle. Energy Transfer Points can be surprisingly tender.

2. Varying the pressure each time you do the massage.

7. Occipital Point Massage

Purpose

1. To stimulate acupressure points located in the occipital region. (The occipital lobes, the primary visual processing centers of the brain, are in a band between your ears in the back lower part of your head.)

2. To relax and reduce neck tension.

REPETITIONS 1 time

TIME 1 - $1\frac{1}{2}$ minutes

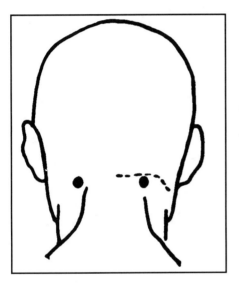

Fig. 15 OCCIPITAL POINT MASSAGE stimulates the acupressure points for vision and also relaxes neck tension.

Instructions

1. Find the acupressure points by following the muscles on either sides of your spine up the back of your neck to where they meet the base of your skull. The points that are tender or sensitive are the ones that you want to massage. (Fig. 15)

2. Apply deep (but not painful) pressure with your fingertips or with the sides of your thumbs for approximately 1 - $1\frac{1}{2}$ minutes.

3. Looking straight ahead, breathe into the pressure. Keep your eyes open and relaxed.

8. Palming

Purpose

To relax tired or strained eyes and restore peace and quiet to your mind.

REPETITIONS --

TIME 1 - $1\frac{1}{2}$ minutes

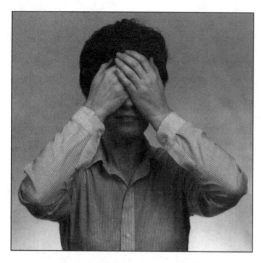

Fig. 16 PALMING is an excellent exercise to relax your eyes and soothe your mind.

Instructions

1. Briskly rub your hands and palms together until they feel warm (15 - 20 seconds).

2. Place your cupped palms over your closed eyes. The fingers of each hand should overlap and rest on the center of your forehead. (Fig. 16)

3. Make sure there is no contact between your palms and your closed eyelids. Also make sure there is enough room between your palms (as they cup your eyes) so that you can breathe easily. Don't create any unnecessary pressure on your face. If your arms get tired, palm resting your elbows on your thighs or on a table.

What to watch for

1. In most cases, seeing sparks, dots of light, or patterns of color are signs that you are releasing mental strain and nervous tension.

2. Seeing blackness with your eyes closed indicates relaxation. As your eyes become more and more relaxed, the black will appear even more black.

Vision Session Three:

Vision Chart Techniques

Vision Session Three, **Vision Chart Techniques**, contains the following series of nine exercises:

1. **Swinging**
2. **Near-To-Far Shifting**
3. **Palming**
4. **Corner-To-Corner Shifting**
5. **Palming**
6. **Eye Stretches**
7. **Palming**
8. **Edging**
9. **Eye Squeezes**

Which vision chart to use

Which vision chart you will use depends on whether you are nearsighted or farsighted or want to improve astigmatism.

If you are nearsighted (have difficulty seeing distant objects), sit or stand as *far away* as you can from the "I Love To See" chart (P. 189) while still being able to read the larger letters (the "I", the "L" in "Love" and the "S" in "See"). Degree of clarity is not important now. An alternative is to use the "I Can See" chart (P. 191) and to sit as *far away* as you can while still being able to read the top three or four lines of the chart (but not the bottom three or four).

Nearsighted people can continue to use the "I Love To See" chart until the small letters around the center design begin to be clear from approximately 20 feet. (At this point you should be able to pass your state's driver's test without glasses.)

If you are farsighted (have trouble seeing near objects), treat the "I Can See" chart as if it were a page out of a magazine and sit as *close to* the chart as you can (20 inches or closer) to be able to read the top three or four lines (but not the bottom three or four). Again, degree of clarity is not important at this time.

Work with this chart until you can read all the lines easily at all distances between six and 20 inches.

If you are both nearsighted and farsighted (use bifocals), select the chart for the first vision problem that you had.

For astigmatism, sit or stand at least four feet from the "I Love To See" chart when doing the Edging exercise (P. 86). With one eye at a time, Edge around the individual bars that make up the circular shapes (two at the top and two at the bottom) on the chart.

Place the vision chart you will be using on the wall so that its center is at eye level. Be sure you are directly in front of the chart. If you choose to do the techniques while standing (which helps to improve posture and balance), make sure the center of the chart is at eye level when you are standing and that you stand directly in front of the chart.

As your vision improves, adjust your distance from the chart accordingly (even during each Vision Session). Nearsighted people will be able to move farther back and farsighted people will be able to move closer and still see with the same or greater degree of clarity; those with astigmatism will be able to see all circles on the chart with equal clarity.

1. Swinging (See Pp. 70-71 for instructions)

REPETITIONS 100

TIME 4 - 5 minutes

2. Near-To-Far Shifting

Purpose

1. To regain flexibility in the muscles that control the movements of your eyes.

2. To improve eye coordination so that your eyes follow the focusing directions from your mind.

3. To develop a balanced use of your eyes.

4. To increase your peripheral awareness.

REPETITIONS 50

TIME $1 - 1\frac{1}{2}$ minutes

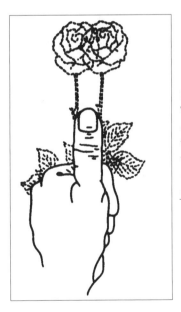

Fig. 17A
When you focus on your finger in the foreground, you'll see two images of the distant target.

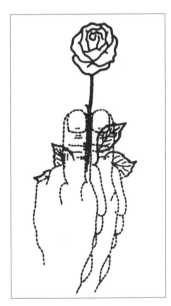

Fig. 17B
When you focus on the distant target, you'll see two images of your thumb.

Instructions

1. As you face the chart, hold your index finger six to 12 inches in front of your eyes. Focus on a small detail of your finger approximately the size of a pinhead. In the background, see the illusion of two charts. (Fig. 17A)

2. Then, in a relaxed manner, shift your focus to the chart to a point the size of a shirt button or smaller. In the foreground, see the illusion of two fingers. (Fig. 17B)

Make sure that your focus goes all the way to the target and rests on the target for a brief moment before you shift your vision back again.

What to watch for

1. If you see only one finger or one chart instead of two make sure both eyes are open and that you're seated directly in front of the chart and that your finger is in front of your nose between you and the spot on the chart at which you're looking.

2. If you still see only one chart or one finger it means that your mind is suppressing the image from one eye. (Suppression is a strained, unnatural state.)

Continued practice should activate the mind's use of both eyes rather quickly. It may take longer than that, but you can speed up the process by issuing a verbal command such as, *"Mind, use both eyes equally."*

3. If you begin to lose the illusion of two charts or two fingers, close your eyes and take a deep breath. Then reopen your eyes, blink lightly, breathe and continue.

4. Initially you may find it easier, more natural and more spontaneous shifting in one direction. As you continue you will develop equal ease, speed and comfort shifting in both directions. Work with the technique until you can shift and focus with your finger three to five inches from your nose.

3. Palming (See P. 78 for instructions)

REPETITIONS --
TIME 30 seconds

4. Corner-To-Corner Shifting

Purpose

1. To promote relaxation and smooth eye movements.
2. To develop central fixation — the ability of the eyes to see one point best.
3. To develop greater control of the focusing mechanisms of your eyes.
4. To isolate eye muscle movement from head movement.
5. To reduce muscular strain and tension in your eyes, neck and head.

4A. Moving your head, nose and eyes

REPETITIONS 10 times (in each direction)
TIME 1 minute

Instructions

1. Imagine a pointer extending from the tip of your nose to the chart.

2. Moving your head, point your nose (the pointer) at each successive corner of the chart using the following four sequences (Figs. 18A - D):

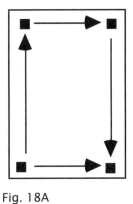 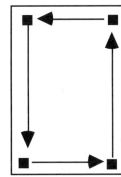 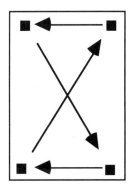

| Fig. 18A | Fig. 18B | Fig. 18C | Fig. 18D |

3. Don't "try to see." Let your eyes follow the movement of your head and nose.

4B. Moving only your eyes

REPETITIONS 10 times (in each direction)
TIME 1 minute

Instructions

1. In the same directions and sequence, move and point only your eyes from corner to corner while keeping your neck, head, forehead and jaw still and relaxed. Again, make sure your head is straight and not tilted.

What to watch for

1. Holding your breath. This indicates undue effort, straining or "trying to see." Keep breathing. And remember to blink regularly, too.

2. Tension in your neck, shoulders or jaw. If you are feeling any, do some Head Rolls to relax. (P. 71)

3. The illusion of movement. When your eyes are moving in a relaxed way, it will seem as if the chart is moving in the opposite direction than your head and eyes (much as the room did when you were swinging). This means that you are moving your eyes in a relaxed way, which is what you want.

5. Palming (See P. 78 for instructions)

REPETITIONS --
TIME 30 seconds

6. Eye Stretches

Purpose

1. To relax, coordinate and tone the six muscles surrounding your eyes.
2. To reduce the pressure in your eyes.

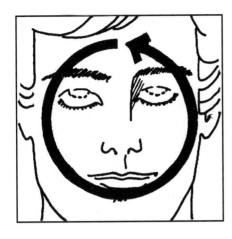

Fig. 19 Rotate your eyes in a circular motion when doing EYE STRETCHES, first clockwise, then counter-clockwise.

REPETITIONS 20 times (in each direction)

TIME 3 minutes

Instructions

1. Close your eyes. Keeping your neck and head still, relax your temples, forehead and your facial muscles. Breathe easily and regularly.

2. Imagine your face to be a clock with your nose at the center. As you stretch your eyes all the way up, you can just barely see the number 12 at the top of this imaginary clock. As you stretch your eyes all the way down, you can barely see the 6 at the bottom.

3. Stretch your eyes as you rotate them in a clockwise direction. Do not strain or force the movements. Repeat for 20 clockwise circles.

4. Change direction and make 20 circles in a counterclockwise direction. (Fig. 19)

Variation

1. To help astigmatism, do Eye Stretches with your head turned to different directions — down, up, halfway to the left and right, or at any angle you choose. Your astigmatism will be helped most by practicing Eye Stretches with your head held in the position in which the eye movements feel most difficult or strained. Practicing in this position until the eye movements are more relaxed and fluid.

What to watch for

1. Your eyes unconsciously jumping out of your control and places of stiffness,

tension or stuckness. Go back over these areas. After a while your stretches will become easier and more fluid and the problem areas will disappear.

2. Holding your breath. Remember, breathe!

3. For variety you can do Eye Stretches with your head facing in any direction (up, down, at an angle, etc.). This may help in situations where astigmatism is present.

7. Palming (See P. 78 for instructions)

REPETITIONS --
TIME 30 seconds

8. Edging

Purpose
1. To develop better coordination between your mind and your eyes so that your eyes converge exactly at the point where you want them to.
2. To sharpen mental concentration.

REPETITIONS --
TIME 4 minutes

Instructions
1. Imagine a pencil extending from the tip of your nose to the chart.

2. While moving both your head and neck, edge around the outline of the objects in your view as if the imaginary pencil were tracing it. (Fig. 20). (Alternatively, you can edge around the outline of any symbol or letter on the vision chart.)

3. Let your eyes follow (rather than lead) the movement of the pencil.

4. Continue for approximately 30 seconds.

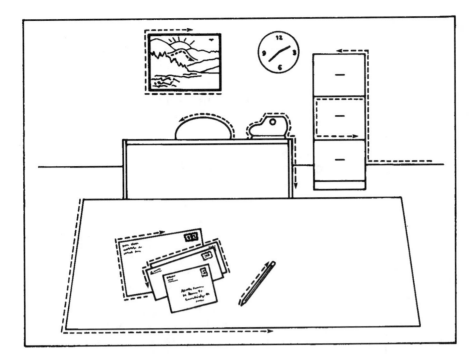

Fig. 20
EDGING helps you develop better eye control and mental concentration.

5. Edge moving only your eyes, Keep your head, temples, facial muscles, neck and shoulders still (and relaxed). Edge in both directions, changing direction often.

6. Continue for approximately 2 minutes.

7. With your eyes closed, "see" in your imagination what you have been edging and — actually moving your closed eyes — edge all the way around in both directions.

8. Continue for approximately 30 seconds.

9. Open your eyes and edge again, moving only your eyes for approximately 1 minute.

What to watch for

1. If your concentration slips your focus will seem to jump or wander past where you're looking. If this happens go back and re-edge the area(s) that you skipped.

2. Sometimes what you are looking at changes. Edge what you see at the present moment — not what you think you should be seeing or what you saw in the last moment.

3. Holding your breath. Remember, breathe!

9. Eye Squeezes

Purpose

1. To increase the circulation and oxygen supply to your eyes and face, thus enervating your visual system.

2. To relax your eye muscles.

3. To break any squinting habits and release any associated tension.

REPETITIONS 2 sets of 5 times each

TIME 1 minute

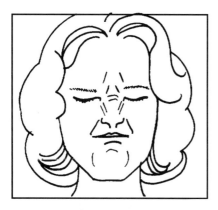

Fig. 21A Begin with a deep inhale as you tighten all the muscles of your face and eyes.

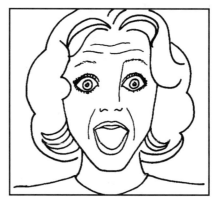

Fig. 21B As you exhale, stretch all the muscles of your face and eyes.

Instructions

1. Inhale deeply, at the same time squeezing your eyes as tightly shut as you can. Squeeze all the muscles in your face, neck and head. Clench your jaw tightly, too.

2. Holding your breath, continue squeezing as tight as you can. (Fig. 21A)

3. Now, exhale quickly, releasing all the tension in your body.

4. Stretch your eyes open wide, open your mouth wide and let out a sigh. (Fig. 21B)

What to watch for

1. Temporary flashes of clear vision. (The key is squeezing tight, letting go quickly and opening your eyes wide.)

2. Sometimes it takes a few moments before your vision becomes clearer. If that's the case, you may want to palm for two or three minutes after doing eye squeezes.

3. Spasms or twitching in your eyelids or your eye muscles. (This is a normal response.)

Vision Session Four:

Mind's Eye Visualization

Vision Session Four, **Mind's Eye Visualization**, consists of only this one visualization.

Purpose

1. To develop the ability to visualize — to produce images with your mind's eye.
2. To encourage the natural coordination between your eyes and your brain/mind.
3. To promote the deep physical and mental relaxation vital to clear vision.

TIME approximately 10 minutes

Instructions

1. Take a deep breath, and as you exhale, let go of any uncomfortable physical sensations... Now, take another deep breath, and as you exhale this time, let go of any discomfort that you might be experiencing on any level, in any part of your body.

2. Begin a regular rhythm of deep, slow and full breathing, relaxing yourself more and more.

3. Guide your imagination through the following visualization:

> In your imagination, leave the room that you are in and go to your special place.

> In this special place you will find yourself outdoors in nature, in the bright sun with mountains and water — maybe a stream, an ocean or a lake.

> Spend some time getting accustomed to being here. Bend down and touch the ground. How does it feel? Notice where you are standing. Are you standing on grass? Is it soft, or are you standing on a hard surface? Become aware of the sensations and textures that you feel underneath your feet.

Go over to the water. Cup some water in your hands and taste it. How does that taste? Is it cool? Is it salty or fresh?

Listen to the sounds around you. What do you hear? The wind rustling in the leaves? Animals scurrying about? Listen to everything that you can hear. And become aware of how sharp and clear your hearing is. You are able to hear the smallest sound from very far away, and you can also hear everything that is happening right near you. Take a moment and listen to all the different sounds that you hear.

Look around now, and the most amazing thing about being here in this place is that wherever you look, everything that you see you're seeing perfectly clearly. You can look off in the distance, to the tops of the mountains, back up close to the ground right beneath your feet, and everywhere in between. And everywhere you look, everything that you see you are seeing perfectly clearly.

And as you see everything perfectly clearly, how do you feel? Notice how your eyes feel, and how your body feels too. Take a moment now to express how you feel as you are seeing everything so clearly and so sharply. You might want to jump up and down, or sing, or dance, or sit in a very peaceful way. Let those feelings of seeing clearly fill you, wash over you and through you. How do you feel as you're seeing everything perfectly clearly?

Continue to look around, because it's amazing, and it's wondrous, to see so much. The colors are so vibrant. You can see the depth and distance; you can look off into the mountains, close up at the ground beneath your feet; and you can see the space in between.

You look off to the left, and notice what's there. And then you look off to the right, and see what's there, too. And you notice that whatever you're looking at, you're seeing it perfectly clearly. And as you're seeing perfectly clearly, you're also feeling all those feelings that you feel when you see this clearly. The clarity, the strength, the peacefulness, and the beauty that's inside and out.

It's just about time to leave. But, before you do, take a final look around, and know that you can come back here anytime that you want to. And every time that you do come back here, everything that you see you will see perfectly clearly and perfectly sharply.

Right now return to the room and keep your eyes closed. Stretch your fingers and wiggle your toes, become aware of your body.

Take a deep breath, and as you sigh on the exhale, become aware of your surroundings. Take one more deep breath, and as you exhale, open your eyes.

Take a deep breath, and slowly open your eyes.

This is the end of the visualization.

What to watch for

1. The scene must include mountains and water, but you can place it anywhere — wherever your imagination takes you. It could be a real place that you've been to or one that you create in your mind for the first time during this visualization.

2. Do whatever you need to do to generate the feeling of "seeing," whether it means pretending, faking it or even having to lie to yourself. It's just another way of using your imagination. Be aware that the depth of your feeling is just as important as your imagination of the scene.

3. If you are farsighted, remember to look at things close up in your imagination — the grains of sand on the beach, the petals of a flower, etc.

4. If you are nearsighted, remember to look at things distant in your imagination — a bird flying overhead, a far-away mountain top, etc.

Vision Session Five:

Spectrum Visualization

Vision Session Five, **Spectrum Visualization**, consists of only this one visualization.

Sensory information travels from your eyes to your brain through your optic nerves. As thick as soda straws, optic nerves meet in the center of your head (directly behind the top of your nose) and continue back to the occipital lobes. It is here where you "see" the world. (See P. 38 for a simplified illustration of the visual routing system.)

Purpose

1. To balance, energize and relax your visual system. To release deep levels of tension (and stress) in your visual system and in your body.
2. To develop and exercise your imagination.

TIME approximately 25 minutes (3 minutes for each color)

Instructions

1. Take a deep breath, and as you exhale, let go of any uncomfortable physical sensations... Now, take another deep breath, and as you exhale this time, let go of any discomfort that you might be experiencing on any level, in any part of your body.

2. Begin a regular rhythm of deep, slow and full breathing, relaxing yourself more and more.

3. Guide your imagination through the following visualization:

> In your imagination, and with your feelings, notice where your left eyelid touches the front of your left eyeball. Now, feel your entire left eyeball, which is about an inch in diameter, and just see if you can become aware of the muscles which surround the left eye. Notice now the rear of the left eyeball, where the optic nerve begins to travel to the very center of your head. The optic nerve is

about the diameter of a straw. From the very center of your head, just imagine the left optic nerve traveling back to the rear of your head and to the left occipital lobe.

And now, move over to the right side and to the rear of your head, and feel the right occipital lobe, and become aware of where the right optic nerve leaves the occipital lobe and travels forward to the very center of your head. Now, just follow the route of the right optic nerve from the center of your head to the rear of your right eye. Feel the muscles that surround the right eyeball, and the right eyeball itself, and now the very front of the right eyeball, where the right eyelid touches it.

Now, in front of your left eyeball, just imagine the very dynamic color of RED. Just feel that RED color begin to flow through your left eyeball into the muscles that surround your left eye, and back to the center of the head, through the left optic nerve, and feel that color RED flow from the center of your head back to the left occipital lobe, and fill it with the color RED. Feel the vibrancy and the warmth of this color as it moves from the left occipital lobe over to the right, filling it, energizing it.

And now it moves forward to the very center of your head again, through the right optic nerve, and forward through the right optic nerve to the rear of your right eyeball. Feel the color RED now fill the right eyeball and the muscles which surround the right eye. Just feel your entire visual routing system filled with the color RED. Feel it flow from your left eyeball all the way through your visual routing system, and coming out the right eyeball, removing any tension and clearing it from your visual system.

Now, just let the color RED go from your imagination, and take a deep breath. And feel the aliveness in your eyes from the color RED.

Now, see the color ORANGE in front of your left eye. And let the color ORANGE fill your left eyeball and the muscles which surround the left eyeball. Let the color ORANGE flow through the left optic nerve to the very center of your head, and from the center of your head back through the optic nerve to the left occipital lobe. Clear, pure ORANGE light fills the left occipital lobe, and spills over to the right side now. And from the right occipital lobe, just see the color ORANGE flowing forward through the right optic nerve to the very center of your head, and from there, forward through the right optic nerve to the rear of the right eyeball, surrounding and filling the right eyeball, and all the muscles which surround it. Just feel the color ORANGE flowing through your entire visual system. Feel it cleanse and purify any tension which might have been there.

Now just let the color ORANGE go, take a nice deep breath.................

CONTINUE WITH EACH OF THE FOLLOWING COLORS IN SEQUENCE: (Spend approximately 3 minutes imagining each color moving through your visual system.)

YELLOW
GREEN
BLUE
PURPLE
WHITE

Take a deep breath, and slowly open your eyes.

This is the end of the visualization.

What to watch for

1. The Spectrum Visualization guides your awareness through your entire visual system — your eyes, the muscles surrounding your eyes, your nerve pathways and your brain.

When asked to imagine color, some people immediately "see" the color vividly in their mind's eye. Some, though, need to repeat the name of the color to themselves, while others need to remember something which they own of that color. Still others instantly associate certain colors with certain feelings (e.g., peacefulness with blue).

2. Discover your own way of doing this visualization within the above script, involving yourself without worrying whether you are "doing it right." For example, some people find it more natural to follow a different route. Others find the route different for different colors and different each time they do the visualization.

Vision Session Six:

Memory Visualization

Vision Session Six, **Memory Visualization**, consists of only this one visualization.

Purpose
1. To release negative images and memories which block your having clearer vision.
2. To reunite the separated parts of your self and develop trust in your intuition.
3. To develop greater self acceptance and self love.

TIME approximately 15 minutes

Instructions
1. Take a deep breath, and as you exhale, let go of any uncomfortable physical sensations...Take another deep breath, and as you exhale this time, let go of any discomfort that you might be experiencing on any level, in any part of your body.

2. Begin a regular rhythm of deep, slow and full breathing, relaxing more and more with every breath.

3. Guide your imagination through the following visualization:

Recall an event that occurred yesterday.

Let that go, and bring to mind an event that occurred a week ago. Any event will do.

Let that go. Now, go back to last winter, and recall an event that occurred around that period of time.

Let that go. Go back now to the year before you first noticed a limitation with your vision. Find yourself standing in front of the house you lived in at that time.

You're about ready to enter into the house, so reach out, grasp the door handle, open the door, and enter into this house that you lived in the year before you first noticed a limitation with your vision.

What is the first room that you enter? What are the colors on the walls? What furniture do you see? Is there a particular scent that always identified this house for you?

Walk through some of the other rooms in this house, noticing the different furniture in the different rooms, noticing those things that made this house *yours*. Perhaps in one of the rooms there was a chair or a sofa that you really liked to sit on. Sit down now; become comfortable. Lean back and relax in this house.

How do you feel as you're back in this environment, in this room?

As you find yourself moving through the different rooms in this house, you're now approaching the doorway to the room that was your bedroom. But don't go in yet — stand in the doorway, and look into the room. Where do you keep your clothes? What color were the walls painted? What are some of the possessions that you have in this room, that made this room *your* room?

As you turn and look through all of the room, your focus moves to the bed. And there, sleeping in the bed, is a person, and that person appears to be you, sleeping there in that bed.

Go over to that person, but don't wake that person up yet. Sit on the edge of the bed, and for a moment, look at that person sleeping there, who appears to be you. And now — gently and quietly, and lovingly — reach forward and wake this person up. Take a moment and look in each other's eyes.

You have come here to speak to this person, and to listen to what this person has to say to you. So, the first question that you'd like to ask this person is "Why am I here to see you?", and listen to what this person has to say.

The next question that you may want to ask this person is "How can you help me?", and listen to what this person has to say.

You may also want to ask this person if there is anything else that they can tell you, and listen to what this person has to say.

Now, thank this person for talking with you, for sharing with you in the way that they have.

But it's not time to leave yet — continue to sit on the edge of the bed, and start to count from one to five. And when you reach five, the person that you both most need to see to help you with your vision will appear at the doorway to your room.

One...Two...Three...Four...Five.

That person is there. Look at that person for a moment and, without saying anything, let that person look into your eyes, as you look into theirs. Communicate through your eyes, without using words. Notice how you're feeling, and also how this person who has come to visit you is feeling.

The first questions you might want to ask this person are "Why have you come here now?" and "What do you have to tell me?" And listen to what this person has to say.

You may want to ask the person if there is anything that he or she can tell you about your vision right now. And listen to what they have to say.

You may want to ask the person if there is anything else that they can tell you now that would be of assistance to you. And, if there is anything, listen to what this person has to say.

Thank this person now for everything that they have told you, for their willingness to take the time, and to express the loving. Thank that person for coming into the room right now.

Turn once again to face that person in the bed — that person who appears to be you, and look into the eyes of this person. Look into the eyes, and speak to each other of the heart, without using words. Express the loving that has always been there, express the caring that has always been there, show the understanding that has always been there.

It's time now to let that person go back to sleep. Lay that person down. You may want to reach over, caress the cheek, or kiss the forehead lightly; tuck the person back to bed.

It's time now for you to leave this house. Walk through any of the rooms that you need to go back to the front door. Exit through the front door, and begin to walk down the street.

But stop — stop for a moment, and as you turn back, see the image of the house disappearing from view. And you know that this is all in the past, and it no longer needs to affect you in any adverse way.

You have taken the learning and the wisdom from this period of your life, and you have gained from it, benefited by it.

The image of the house completely disappears from view. You find yourself becoming aware of your body, becoming aware of the surroundings.

Wiggle your hands, stretch your fingers. Take a deep breath, exhale and open your eyes.

This is the end of the visualization.

What to watch for

1. It is not important to accurately remember every detail of the house you visit. Instead, let the memories, thoughts, feelings and images surface naturally. Take what's there. "Trying to remember" blocks the intuitive process.

2. In your daily life look for ways to apply the messages that you receive during this visualization.

3. Let your imagination go. You'll probably find that each time you do the visualization your experience and your memories will be different.

4. Remember that the people you see — your younger self and the visitor — are different aspects of your own self.

5. The more you do the Memory Visualization, the clearer the channel will become between your conscious and intuitive selves.

CHAPTER FIFTEEN

HOW TO USE
THE FIRST STAGE SCHEDULE

"Life can only be understood looking backwards; but it must be lived looking forwards."

—Søren Kierkegaard, l9th century philosopher

The FIRST STAGE is an 8-week schedule during which you will practice one of the Six Vision Sessions on each practice day. The schedule that begins on P. 106 tells you which Vision Session to do on each day.

On the first day of the 8-week schedule complete Part A of **THE FIRST STAGE** report (Pp. 195 - 196). On the last day, complete Parts B & C. Remove the report (or copy it) and mail it back to the Cambridge Institute for Better Vision.

At the top of the page of each week's schedule is a series of boxes. On each practice day, acknowledge with a check mark (in the appropriate daily box) that you've completed that day's training and write (in the tiny box in the right-hand corner of the daily box) the number of hours you went without glasses or contacts.

Once a week, at the last session, complete the weekly review questions. You will also be asked to reflect on a positive thought — a vision affirmation — on a daily basis.

During **THE FIRST STAGE** you will be asked to do all six Vision Sessions a number of times. Some of the Sessions may seem to be directly related to your eyesight while others, at first, may seem not to be.

Please don't make the mistake of only doing parts because you think you know what to do to improve your vision. Each technique and visualization plays an integral role in your vision improvement. If you only use parts you will not realize the maximum benefits that you could and you might not see any improvement at all. It is important to complete all the parts.

It's easy to be dissatisfied with your vision without glasses — after all, that's what motivated you to improve — but the way to get the most results is to accept what you can see every step of the way.

Expect that your feelings about your vision will fluctuate. As well as feeling positive and hopeful, there may be times when you lack enthusiasm or feel discouraged. This is all part of releasing emotional stress and readjusting to clear vision. When such feelings surface, use them as reminders of your commitment to seeing clearly. Keep your perspective. Remember where you are with your vision and where you want to be.

THE FIRST STAGE schedule is designed so that at the same time as you practice the techniques and visualizations you will also learn to identify and clear up any difficulties you encounter along the way.

Your attitude during these eight weeks also will make a difference. Improving your vision has a dramatic effect on many levels of consciousness. You must develop an emotional and mental willingness to look honestly, openly and clearly. This is the inner foundation you need to allow yourself to benefit the most from the techniques.

Positive thought of the week

There is a positive thought for each week that we strongly suggest you use. Simply, the idea is to bring this vision affirmation into your everyday awareness. Say it out loud. Repeat it to yourself. Keep it in your consciousness.

This positive thought can be used to replace the limiting thoughts that you may have about your vision. Since your subconscious listens to what you think and to what it has heard you repeat over the years, it is important to start changing the message inside of you to a positive one. Repeating the positive thought trains your mind to focus on what you want — in this case, **Better Vision**.

It is not necessary to believe the positive thought. Say it even if you don't believe it. By repeating the positive thought you will begin to replace the old subconscious (negative) habit of not seeing with a new conscious (positive) habit of wanting to see more clearly. (See **Using Affirmations For Better Vision**, Pp. 167 - 169.)

If you miss a practice session

The seventh day of each week is a rest day. It is better for you to take the break you deserve after six straight days than not. But if you miss a day during the week you can stay on track by using the free day as a make-up day.

Also, if for some reason you need to stop following the schedule for an extended period of time, you can either pick up where you left off or start over at the beginning again.

It is possible to derive some benefit by using the techniques and visualizations less frequently than every day. You may find temporary relief from eyestrain and headaches, gain some needed relaxation, and relieve the visual and body stress that you pick up daily, but remember — only regular and consistent practice will bring you the most satisfying and noticeable results.

If you want to do more

If you want to do more in a day than the scheduled practice, do so. Just follow these suggestions:

1. Do not jump ahead in the schedule.

2. Balance each day's practice between techniques and visualizations. This means that if the schedule calls for a series of techniques and you want to do more, practice a visualization to which you have already been introduced.

3. We also highly recommend doing the Affirmation Writing Exercise (Pp. 168 - 169) on a regular — if not daily — basis.

CHAPTER SIXTEEN

The First Stage Schedule: Day By Day

DAY 1	DAY 2	DAY 3	DAY 4	DAY 5	DAY 6	DAY 7

WEEK 1

POSITIVE THOUGHT OF THE WEEK:
MY EYES ARE GOOD, MY EYES ARE NORMAL

SCHEDULE:

DAY 1 **COMPLETE PART A of THE FIRST STAGE REPORT**
(Pp. 195 - 196)

DAY 2 **FUSION STRING TECHNIQUE**
(VISION SESSION 1: Pp. 64 - 68)

DAY 3 **MIND'S EYE VISUALIZATION**
(VISION SESSION 4: Pp. 90 - 92)

DAY 4 **FUSION STRING TECHNIQUE**
(VISION SESSION 1: Pp. 64 - 68)

DAY 5 **FUSION STRING TECHNIQUE**
(VISION SESSION 1: Pp. 64 - 68)

DAY 6 **MIND'S EYE VISUALIZATION**
(VISION SESSION 4: Pp. 90 - 92)
WEEKLY REVIEW

DAY 7 **OFF,** no practice.

WEEKLY REVIEW:

1. What did you accomplish with the Fusion String at the end of the week that you couldn't do at the beginning?

2. What were the most noticeable physical and/or emotional affects that you experienced working with the Fusion String?

3. What are your feelings when you imagine yourself having clear vision?

4. What in your personality or behavior prevents you from expressing these feelings more now in your daily life?

5. What did you learn about yourself and your vision this week?

6. How can you focus more fully on next week's positive thought?

7. List at least 10 positive experiences — changes in attitude, feeling, relaxation, acuity, etc. — you had this week with your vision.

DAY 1	DAY 2	DAY 3	DAY 4	DAY 5	DAY 6	DAY 7

WEEK 2

POSITIVE THOUGHT OF THE WEEK:
I AM ACCEPTING MY VISION THE WAY IT IS

SCHEDULE:

DAY 1 **FUSION STRING TECHNIQUE**
(*VISION SESSION 1: Pp. 64 - 68*)

DAY 2 **FUSION STRING TECHNIQUE**
(*VISION SESSION 1: Pp. 64 - 68*)

DAY 3 **MIND'S EYE VISUALIZATION**
(*VISION SESSION 4: Pp. 90 - 92*) (*twice during the day*)

DAY 4 **MIND'S EYE VISUALIZATION**
(*VISION SESSION 4: Pp. 90 - 92*) (*twice during the day*)

DAY 5 **FUSION STRING TECHNIQUE**
(*VISION SESSION 1: Pp. 64 - 68*)

DAY 6 **MIND'S EYE VISUALIZATION**
(*VISION SESSION 4: Pp. 90 - 92*) (*once, before the review*)
WEEKLY REVIEW

DAY 7 **OFF**, no practice.

WEEKLY REVIEW:

1. What did you accomplish with the Fusion String this week?

2. What physical or emotional affects did you experience working with the Fusion String?

3. What changes have you noticed in your vision either before, during or after your Fusion String practice sessions?

4. Are there any improvements that you can make to your practice area to make it more comfortable? More effective?

5. What did you learn about yourself and your vision this week?

6. List any new activities that you will be able to do without your glasses/contact lenses in the coming week.

7. List at least 10 positive experiences you had this week with your vision.

DAY 1	DAY 2	DAY 3	DAY 4	DAY 5	DAY 6	DAY 7

WEEK 3

POSITIVE THOUGHT OF THE WEEK:
I AM RELEASING ALL BARRIERS TO CLEAR VISION

SCHEDULE:

DAY 1   **SELF MASSAGE TECHNIQUE**
           (VISION SESSION 2: Pp. 69 - 78)

DAY 2   **SPECTRUM VISUALIZATION**
           (VISION SESSION 5: Pp. 93 - 96)

DAY 3   **FUSION STRING TECHNIQUE**
           (VISION SESSION 1: Pp. 64 - 68)

DAY 4   **SELF MASSAGE TECHNIQUE**
           (VISION SESSION 2: Pp. 69 - 78)

DAY 5   **SPECTRUM VISUALIZATION**
           (VISION SESSION 5: Pp. 93 - 96)

DAY 6   **SELF MASSAGE TECHNIQUE**
           (VISION SESSION 2: Pp. 69 - 78)
           WEEKLY REVIEW

DAY 7   **OFF,** no practice.

WEEKLY REVIEW:

1. What feelings or thoughts were you aware of when you touched your eyes?

2. Describe your experiences with the Spectrum Visualization.

3. In what new areas of your body are you now feeling tension and/or relaxation? Any other physical effects?

4. What thoughts and feelings did you notice this week related to your vision practice?

5. List at least 10 positive experiences you had this week with your vision.

(Complete these sentences)

6. In order to have clear vision, the personal habits that I would need to change are

7. If I had clear vision, the feelings that I would have are

DAY 1	DAY 2	DAY 3	DAY 4	DAY 5	DAY 6	DAY 7

WEEK 4

POSITIVE THOUGHT OF THE WEEK:
I AM ALWAYS NOTICING WHAT I CAN SEE

SCHEDULE:

DAY 1   **FUSION STRING TECHNIQUE**
            (VISION SESSION 1: Pp. 64 - 68)

DAY 2   **SELF MASSAGE TECHNIQUE**
            (VISION SESSION 2: Pp. 69 - 78)

DAY 3   **SPECTRUM VISUALIZATION**
            (VISION SESSION 5: Pp. 93 - 96)

DAY 4   **FUSION STRING TECHNIQUE**
            (VISION SESSION 1: Pp. 64 - 68)

DAY 5   **SELF MASSAGE TECHNIQUE**
            (VISION SESSION 2: Pp. 69 - 78)

DAY 6   **MIND'S EYE VISUALIZATION**
            (VISION SESSION 4: Pp. 90 - 92) (once, before the review)
            WEEKLY REVIEW

DAY 7   **OFF,** no practice.

WEEKLY REVIEW:

1. What was different about your vision or about your relationship to your vision this week?

2. List at least three major events that occurred in your life in the year before you first noticed a limitation in your vision.

3. Briefly describe 10 early (childhood) memories.

4. What changes in your vision are you noticing outdoors?

5. List at least 10 positive qualities about yourself.

6. List at least 10 qualities about yourself that you would like to change.

7. List any new activities that you will do without glasses in the coming week.

DAY 1	DAY 2	DAY 3	DAY 4	DAY 5	DAY 6	DAY 7

WEEK 5

POSITIVE THOUGHT OF THE WEEK:
I AM TRUSTING WHAT I SEE

SCHEDULE:

DAY 1   **FUSION STRING TECHNIQUE**

       (VISION SESSION 1: Pp. 64 - 68)

DAY 2   **SPECTRUM VISUALIZATION**

       (VISION SESSION 5: Pp. 93 - 96)

DAY 3   **VISION CHART TECHNIQUE**

       (VISION SESSION 3: Pp. 79 - 89)

DAY 4   **MIND'S EYE VISUALIZATION**

       (VISION SESSION 4: Pp. 90 - 92) (twice during the day)

DAY 5   **MEMORY VISUALIZATION**

       (VISION SESSION 6: Pp. 97 - 101)

DAY 6   **WEEKLY REVIEW**

DAY 7   **OFF,** no practice.

WEEKLY REVIEW:

1. What feelings were evoked during the Memory Visualization?

2. What were the messages that your younger self and your visitor told you?

3. In what ways have your attitudes or feelings about yourself (or others) changed as a result of the Memory Visualization?

4. What changes did you notice while you were working with the vision chart?

(Complete this sentence)
5. The emotional benefits that I get from **not** seeing clearly are

(Complete this sentence)
6. The parts of myself that I don't want to see are

7. Describe your responses (positive or negative) to this week's positive thought.

DAY 1	DAY 2	DAY 3	DAY 4	DAY 5	DAY 6	DAY 7

WEEK 6

POSITIVE THOUGHT OF THE WEEK:
I AM ALLOWING MY VISION TO CLEAR

SCHEDULE:

DAY 1   **FUSION STRING TECHNIQUE**
(VISION SESSION 1: Pp. 64 - 68)

DAY 2   **VISION CHART TECHNIQUE**
(VISION SESSION 3: Pp. 79 - 89)

DAY 3   **SPECTRUM VISUALIZATION**
(VISION SESSION 5: Pp. 93 - 96)

DAY 4   **VISION CHART TECHNIQUE**
(VISION SESSION 3: Pp. 79 - 89)

DAY 5   **MEMORY VISUALIZATION**
(VISION SESSION 6: Pp. 97 - 101)

DAY 6   **WEEKLY REVIEW**

DAY 7   **OFF,** no practice.

WEEKLY REVIEW:

1. What changes have you noticed during or after working with the vision chart? Have you moved your chair?

2. During this week's Memory Visualization what messages did you receive from your younger self and your visitor?

3. What changes have there been in your awareness of your vision?

4. What can you see now that you could not see before you started The Program? (List all vision changes, no matter how small or slight.)

5. List at least 10 positive experiences you had this week with your vision.

(Complete these sentences)

6. As I see more clearly, the parts of myself that I would like to express more are

7. The specific areas of my life, my self and my relationships that I would like to see more clearly are

DAY 1	DAY 2	DAY 3	DAY 4	DAY 5	DAY 6	DAY 7

WEEK 7

POSITIVE THOUGHT OF THE WEEK:
I AM NOW ENJOYING EVERYTHING I SEE

SCHEDULE:

DAY 1   **SELF MASSAGE TECHNIQUE**
(*VISION SESSION 2: Pp. 69 - 78*)

DAY 2   **SPECTRUM VISUALIZATION**
(*VISION SESSION 5: Pp. 93 - 96*)

DAY 3   **VISION CHART TECHNIQUE**
(*VISION SESSION 3: Pp. 79 - 89*)

DAY 4   **VISION CHART TECHNIQUE**
(*VISION SESSION 3: Pp. 79 - 89*)

DAY 5   **VISION CHART TECHNIQUE**
(*VISION SESSION 3: Pp. 79 - 89*)

DAY 6   **MIND'S EYE VISUALIZATION**
(*VISION SESSION 4: Pp. 90 - 92*) (*once, before the review*)
WEEKLY REVIEW

DAY 7   **OFF,** no practice.

WEEKLY REVIEW:

1. What changes have you noticed working with the vision chart this week?

2. Did you observe yourself looking into the "blur zone" this week? If yes, what were your responses?

3. List any new activities that you will do without your glasses/contact lenses in the coming week.

4. What Program techniques produce immediate noticeable vision improvement for you?

5. Where are you now feeling tension in your body?

6. What could you do to relax these areas? Be specific.

7. List at least 10 positive experiences you had this week with your vision.

DAY 1	DAY 2	DAY 3	DAY 4	DAY 5	DAY 6	DAY 7

WEEK 8

POSITIVE THOUGHT OF THE WEEK:
MY VISION IS ALWAYS IMPROVING

SCHEDULE:

DAY 1   **FUSION STRING TECHNIQUE**
          (VISION SESSION 1: Pp. 64 - 68)

DAY 2   **SPECTRUM VISUALIZATION**
          (VISION SESSION 5: Pp. 93 - 96)

DAY 3   **VISION CHART TECHNIQUE**
          (VISION SESSION 3: Pp. 79 - 89)

DAY 4   **MEMORY VISUALIZATION**
          (VISION SESSION 6: Pp. 97 - 101)

DAY 5   **SELF MASSAGE TECHNIQUE**
          (VISION SESSION 2: Pp. 69 - 78)

DAY 6   **MIND'S EYE VISUALIZATION**
          (VISION SESSION 4: Pp. 90 - 92)
          WEEKLY REVIEW

DAY 7   **COMPLETE PARTS B & C OF THE FIRST STAGE REPORT**
          (Pp. 196 - 198)

WEEKLY REVIEW:

1. What significant changes in your vision are you (or have you been) noticing during your daily life?

2. How can you become more open and accepting of yourself and others?

3. When do you experience temporary improvement in your vision?

4. Has your ability to visualize changed during THE FIRST STAGE?

5. List at least 10 positive experiences you had this week with your vision.

(Complete the next two sentences)
6. If I had clear vision I would

7. The ways that I can continue improving my vision are

PART 4:

THE
SECOND STAGE

CHAPTER SEVENTEEN

WHAT'S NEXT AFTER THE FIRST STAGE?

Congratulations on completing THE FIRST STAGE 8-week schedule! THE FIRST STAGE is your first step towards **Better Vision**. As you continue working on your vision you can expect further improvement.

If you are wondering what to do next, here are some options to consider:

1. Continue practicing using the schedule from week 8 of THE FIRST STAGE.

2. Create your own practice schedule using the techniques and visualizations that were the most challenging and effective. Generally speaking, those techniques and visualizations that are still difficult or challenging for you are also the ones that will be most beneficial.

3. Work with a behavioral optometrist in your area who offers a program of vision training/therapy. The Cambridge Institute (508-887-3883) may be able to assist you in finding one.

4. Use any of the advanced techniques and visualizations contained in THE SECOND STAGE. They build on the basic principles that you have been introduced to and allow you to do deeper work on the physical, mental and emotional levels. Combine these new techniques and visualizations with those that you will continue to use from THE FIRST STAGE.

5. Obtain your own **Personalized Vision Program** from Martin Sussman. Your **Personalized Vision Program** gives you a customized schedule that contains only those techniques and visualizations that are best for you. Your own program will probably contain techniques and visualizations and special variations that you need that aren't in this book. Call 508-887-3883.

6. Add any of the audiotapes, books and nutritional supplements listed in this Appendix to your daily schedule. (Pp. 199 - 202)

Whichever steps you choose, we encourage and support you to continue to work towards having the clearest vision you possibly can. Contact the Cambridge Institute whenever you have any questions, need more information, want additional support or want to tell us about your successes!

CHAPTER EIGHTEEN

ADVANCED TECHNIQUES AND VISUALIZATIONS

This section contains new techniques and visualizations that you can add to your practice program. Experiment with all of them and then choose which you would like to use regularly. Remember that those that are most difficult or challenging or those that you tend to resist are usually the ones that will bring you the most value and improvement.

The techniques and visualizations of **THE SECOND STAGE** are:

1. **Balance And Coordination Exercises**
2. **Developing The Inner Seer**
3. **Exploring Your "Blur Zone"**
4. **Letting Go Of Visual Tension**
5. **Peripheral And Fusion Awareness**
6. **Peripheral Awareness Exercises**
7. **Unlocking Your Memory**
8. **Vision Rock**
9. **Visual And Muscular Flexibility**

1. Balance And Coordination Exercises

These three exercises are particularly helpful for those who have a difference between the two eyes. The greater the difference, the more valuable these exercises will be. Imbalances between the two eyes are often tied to imbalances in the body, as well as problems with coordination and depth perception. When an imbalance is present, each eye may represent a different aspect of consciousness or a different set of feelings. Gaining greater eye balance and coordination often reflects a greater inner balancing and harmony.

Purpose

1. To encourage the two sides of the body and brain to work together.
2. To support convergence and binocularity skills.
3. To develop greater coordination and visual balance.

1A. Hand/Foot Touch

REPETITIONS 5 sets of 30 times each
TIME 8 minutes

Instructions

1. Stand with your feet together, arms at your side, eyes open, looking straight ahead.

2. Bend your left leg up behind you until your lower leg is parallel to the floor with your toes pointing down. At the same time as you bend your knee, reach behind you with your *right* hand and touch your *left* heel.

3. Return to the starting position in 1.

4. Repeat with your *right* leg and *left* hand.

5. Repeat steps 1 - 5 thirty times. At the correct speed, 30 repetitions should take about 1 minute.

6. Do this 1-minute routine five times, taking a brief rest between each set. When resting, stand with your feet together and your weight distributed equally on both feet. Face straight ahead and keep both eyes closed.

What to watch for
1. Look straight ahead as you reach behind with your hand. Do not turn your head to look at your foot.

Variations
When you can easily do the above, then practice with these variations in this sequence: When variation 1 becomes easy, proceed to 2, then 3, etc.

1. Count out loud, from 1 to 30, counting the next number at the same time as you touch your *right* hand to your *left* foot.

2. Count out loud from 1 to 30, counting the next number at the same time as you touch your *left* hand to your *right* foot.

3. Count out loud by fours, counting the next number at the same time as you touch your *right* hand to your *left* foot.

4. Count out loud by fours, counting the next number at the same time as you touch your *left* hand to your *right* foot.

5. Say your first name out loud *every other time* you touch your *right* foot with your *left* hand, and say your last name out loud *every third time* you touch your *left* foot with your *right* hand.

6. Say your first name out loud *every other time* you touch your *left* foot, and say your last name out loud *every third time* you touch your *right* foot.

1B. Rub Your Tummy/Pat Your Head

This one may sound silly, but it really helps. Sure you know how to do it, but you've probably never knew that it could be used as a vision exercise!

REPETITIONS --
TIME 2 minutes

Instructions

1. First, rub in a clockwise circle on your stomach with your right hand while you are patting your head with your left hand.

2. Switch hands and repeat.

3. Either step 1 or step 2 will be harder for you to do in a smooth manner. Practice whichever is harder. Also, make sure you alternate rubbing both your stomach and your head in clockwise and counter-clockwise directions.

4. Continue for 2 minutes, or until you are able to rhythmically make the movements in a coordinated way.

Variations

1. Count from 1 to 100 as you rub and pat. Maintain rhythm and coordination.

2. Recite a favorite poem or read out loud as you rub and pat.

1C. Walking The Line

REPETITIONS 10 times
TIME 5 - 6 minutes

Instructions

1. Cover your right eye with an eye patch. Keep the covered eye open. Stand with your feet together.

2. Hold your index finger 6 - 8 inches in front of your eyes.

3. Focus on your index finger as you walk forward 10 paces in a straight line, *touching heel to toe* on each step.

4. Continue focusing on your finger as you walk backwards 10 paces in a straight line, *touching toe to heel* on each step.

5. Walk back and forth along this line 10 times.

6. Repeat with left eye covered.

Variations

1. Rotate your finger (and keep focused on it) in a circle in front of your eyes as you walk back and forth. Alternate rotating your finger clockwise and counter-clockwise.

2. Walk back and forth with your eyes closed.

2. Developing The Inner Seer

Purpose

1. To develop your inner willingness to see clearly.

2. To surface and release emotional and subconscious barriers to seeing.

REPETITIONS --

TIME as needed

Instructions

1. Make a list of those things in your life that you do not want to see, are avoiding, denying, pretending are not there, or are hoping will go away. These could be a situation, a feeling, a part of yourself, or another person or relationship. Be honest. This list is for you only — keep it confidential. (Making a truly complete list could be overwhelming. At first, you might want to limit it to 10 important items.)

2. One at a time, take each item on the list and write down everything about it that you have been avoiding. Be specific and complete. Is there a negative outcome that is feared? Are you avoiding a particular feeling(s)? Are you resisting what your intuition is telling you? etc., etc. Go deeper and deeper, looking for the most crucial, underlying aspect.

3. Write down how you would benefit by seeing it clearly and dealing with it directly. What is the positive result that would follow? What positive qualities in yourself would you have to draw on or develop in order to see it clearly?

4. For each item, list the action steps that you can take to achieve the positive outcome.

5. Start taking those steps now.

Variation

1. Do this technique through the eyes of your younger self — the person that you were during your **Transitional Period** (P. 44) — the year or two before you first noticed a limitation in your vision.

2. Write down the steps that you could have taken then, but didn't.

3. Exploring Your "Blur Zone"

The "blur zone" is that part of your visual field that you do not now see clearly without glasses. There is a visual boundary between your "blur zone'" and your "clear zone".

For nearsighted people, the blur zone begins about one or two feet away. Many people who became nearsighted early in life received negative messages about exploring the world from one or both parents and need to give themselves permission to see and explore without fear or pressure.

For farsighted people, the blur zone is usually within arm's length. A farsighted person sees better by pushing things farther away. This stance of "pushing away" is often mirrored in the personality — through fear of intimacy and of receiving, for example.

People tend not to look into the "blur zone" without glasses or lenses because they can't see it clearly and so they think, *"why bother to look?"* Or they don't have the patience to take the time and look. These negative, limiting tendencies create a downward spiral — the less you look, the less you see. These attitudes also tend to negatively interfere with the brain/eye connection.

Even if what you are seeing is not clear, it is extremely helpful to explore your blur zone.

Purpose
1. To stretch your vision out of its clear zone and stimulate the brain/eye connection.
2. To encourage you to explore your visual world.

REPETITIONS --
TIME 15 - 20 minutes (or longer)

Instructions

1. If you are nearsighted, choose a distant view (i.e., mountains, open field, long highway). If you are farsighted, choose a view within arm's length (a magazine page, photograph, newspaper). It is best if your view has a variety of shapes and colors.

2. Explore this scene and practice any or all of the techniques that you know: Edging, Near-to-Far Shifting, Corner-to-Corner Shifting, Blinking, Peripheral Awareness, etc.

What to watch for

1. Do not strain to see better or more clearly. Instead, relax and accept what you are seeing, regardless of the degree of clarity. Breathe, stay relaxed and blink regularly.

2. Look for differences in what you are seeing. It may be a "blur zone", but the more you look and the more you see, the more distinction and difference you will notice. Looking for differences encourages the visual centers of the brain to become re-involved in seeing.

3. Practice seeing with the eyes of a child. Don't compare what you are seeing to how you think it should look. Instead, imagine that you are seeing everything for the very first time. This attitude encourages the same kind of excitement and curiosity with which a child might see the world.

4. Letting Go Of Visual Tension

Purpose

1. To relax your body, your extra-ocular muscles and your ciliary muscles.

2. To use the mind to restore flexibility and tone to your ciliary muscles and your lens.

3. To bring new awareness to your visual system.

REPETITIONS --

TIME 20 - 30 minutes

The muscles of the ciliary body work together to change the curvature of the lens and thereby adjust the focusing power of your eyes. (Re-read **How The Eyes Work** [Pp. 16 - 19].)

Instructions

1. Take a deep breath, and as you exhale, let go of any uncomfortable physical sensations... Now, take another deep breath, and as you exhale this time, let go of any discomfort that you might be experiencing on any level, in any part of your body.

2. Begin a regular rhythm of deep, slow and full breathing, relaxing yourself more and more.

3. Guide your imagination through the following visualization:

> Let your mind come to rest on your breathing. Become aware of your breathing as you inhale and exhale. Feel the rise and fall of your chest as your breath moves in and out.
>
> Become aware of your body as it is supported by the surface on which you are sitting. Feel the different places that your body touches this surface and also feel the temperature in your hands and the temperature of your feet.
>
> And as you feel these sensations, also become aware of all the other sensations that you may be experiencing that let you know that you're becoming more comfortable, that you are relaxing, and that there is a growing sense of inner peacefulness and calm.

Bring your awareness to both of your feet and to the muscles and the bones of your feet, and allow your feet to relax. Allow this relaxation to expand so that it encompasses your ankles, the muscles and bones of your ankles, your calves, your shins, the muscles and bones of your knees and your thighs. Feel this relaxation move through your legs — inside, to their very core and outside, to the very edges of your skin.

Allow this growing sense of relaxation to travel upward and fill your pelvic region and all the muscles and bones of your pelvis, and all the organs situated in this area of your body. Let this area of your body be enveloped by the relaxation that started at the bottom of your feet and has risen and moved upward, enveloping your feet, your legs, your knees, your thighs, your pelvis. Allow this feeling to continue to rise so that you feel your lower torso, the muscles of your lower back and the base of your spine all relax as any remaining tension disappears, leaving only a deeper and deeper feeling of relaxation.

And as this relaxed feeling grows and expands, let it fill all the organs and all the muscles of your solar plexus region, the area of your middle back, all the muscles and organs in this area of your body. Let the tension melt away, and let your relaxation continue to grow and expand and allow it to surround and fill your lungs, your chest and your diaphragm.

Allow your breathing to become even more effortless, natural and relaxed. Feel your shoulder blades and the muscles of your shoulders let go as all the tension falls away. Allow the relaxation to rise and feel your neck relax, feel your throat, the back of your head and the muscles of your jaw and your mouth let go and relax.

Let the muscles of your cheeks relax. Feel your forehead and your temples relax and let go. Feel your eyelids and allow them to relax. Become aware of the contact that your inner eyelids make with the surface of your eyes. Feel that contact, both on your left eye and on your right. And imagine that your eyes — both right and left — are becoming softer, that any hardness is disappearing and your eyes are becoming as soft as a cloud or as light as a helium-filled balloon...as weightless as can be.

Imagine that the six muscles that surround the eyes, the six extra-ocular muscles, are also relaxing, that they are letting go as they need to let go, and the muscles that need to unwind are unwinding, and those that need more tone are adjusting and gaining more tone.

And if you have been nearsighted, imagine that the oblique muscles which surround each eye are unwinding, much as a spring might unwind, becoming looser, softer and lighter, relieving some of the pressure, and your eyes are also feeling softer and lighter, and are letting go, your eyes are returning to their most natural and perfect shape as you simply continue to relax.

Imagine that the recti muscles, which extend from the front to the back of each eye , are adjusting and gaining more tone. Let the recti muscles become more involved in the process of seeing.

And if you have been farsighted, imagine that the recti muscles are relaxing, letting go, and they are letting the eyes return to their natural and more perfect state. And imagine, if you've been farsighted, that the oblique muscles which surround the eyes are developing more tone and doing their part in allowing the eye to return to its perfect shape.

Let the fluid that fills the eye become lighter and let it help in returning the eyes to the perfect and natural shape that will allow you to have clear vision, the clearest vision that you can possibly have. Let the muscles of both eyes return to their natural balance so those that need tone are regaining that tone and those that need to relax are relaxing.

And problems that you once had in seeing clearly at any distance are disappearing, and all the changes that your body, your mind and your eyes need to make are being made, and your vision is returning to its clearest state, and you recognize, and so does your unconscious mind, that you have the ability to see with a sharp focus. You can see in an easy and relaxed way.

And the six extra-ocular muscles of the right eye and the left eye are working together in complete harmony, in perfect balance, adjusting effortlessly and easily letting your eyes and your mind see objects at every distance clearly and in sharp focus.

Any astigmatism that you once had is disappearing as well, and the cornea of both eyes is returning to a natural, original and perfect shape, effortlessly and easily.

And as these muscles continue returning to their natural state of balance, bring your awareness to the focusing lens of the eyes and become aware of the ciliary body of muscles that change and control the shape of the lens.

If you have been nearsighted, imagine that the lens is becoming flatter by the action of the muscles that surround it, and there is less of a bulge in the lens from front to back, and as you imagine this, it allows you to bring objects in the distance into focus easily and effortlessly.

If you have been farsighted, imagine that the lens is bulging more from front to back, that the muscles that surround the lens work in the way they need to, bringing close-up objects into focus.

Imagine the muscles that surround the lens are applying more pressure equally around the diameter of the lens.

Allow your unconscious to make all the changes that it knows need to be made so that you will see as much as you can see as clearly as possible. Simply imagine that your entire visual system is regaining all the flexibility, tone and relaxation that it needs to have exactly the kind of vision that you want to have.

Sense that the muscles of the ciliary body are returning to their natural balance and their natural interplay. And this natural harmony and balance produce clear vision at every distance. Let any remaining tension dissolve and disappear, let it simply drain away from you, drain away from your eyes and the muscles of your eyes, leaving your eyes, your mind, your body and your entire visual system in perfect balance with perfect functioning.

And know that as you are going through the future days and weeks that even when you're not thinking about your eyes or your visual system at all, they are returning to a state of perfect harmony, regaining flexibility, tone, balance and clarity, and you will have clearer and clearer vision, day after day.

Take a deep breath, and slowly open your eyes.

This is the end of the visualization.

5. Peripheral And Fusion Awareness

You are ready to do this exercise only if you can answer YES to all three of these questions:

1. Hold one finger approximately 6 inches directly in front of your nose. Look at an object at least 15 feet away. As you keep focused on the distant object, do you see two images of your finger in the foreground?

2. Focus directly on your finger. Do you see two images of the distant object in the background?

3. As you keep your finger 6 inches from you, hold one finger of the other hand behind the first, approximately 15 inches from your eyes. Look at the finger farthest from you. As you stay focused on that finger, can you see two images of the closer finger in the foreground?

If you answer NO to any of these questions, go back and practice these exercises: **Fusion String Technique** (Pp. 64 - 68), **Near-to-Far Shifting** (Pp. 81 - 82) and **Spectrum Visualization** (Pp. 93 - 96).

Purpose
1. To increase the balance and coordination between the mind and the eyes.
2. To increase the balance between peripheral and central vision.
3. To further awaken the mental aspects of vision.
4. To develop greater convergence and divergence abilities.
5. To release muscular tension and restore flexibility.

REPETITIONS 16 times
TIME 20 minutes
MATERIALS NEEDED Peripheral and Fusion Chart (P. 193)

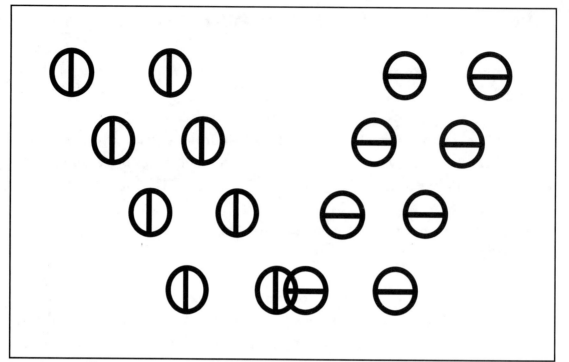

Fig. 22A   You'll see two images of the chart when you look at the wall through the cut-out.

Instructions (Part 1)

1. Sit 10 - 15 feet from a wall.

2. Hold the Peripheral and Fusion Chart approximately 6 inches in front of you at eye level and look at the wall through the cut-out on the chart.

3. In the foreground, you should see two images of the chart. (Fig. 22A)

4. Hold the chart so that row 1 is slightly below eye level.

5. As you continue to look at the wall, adjust your vision so that the center two circles on Row 1 overlap to form a cross. (Fig. 22B)

6. Hold this overlapped image for 20 seconds.

7. Close your eyes and rest for 15 - 20 seconds.

8. Repeat again with the same row.

9. Repeat steps 5 - 8 with each of the three other rows.

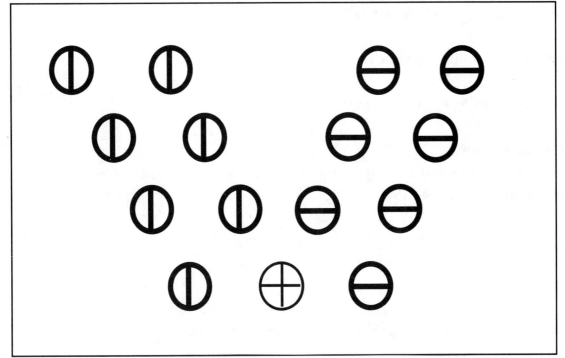

Fig. 22B   When you adjust your vision correctly, two images on the first row will overlap into one, creating a circle containing a cross.

Instructions (Part 2)

1. Attach the Peripheral and Fusion Chart to the wall at eye level. Sit or stand 18 - 20 inches from the Chart.

2. Hold your finger approximately 6 inches in front of you slightly below Row 1, with the Chart in the background.

3. As you focus directly on your finger, notice the double image of the Chart in the background.

4. Slowly move your finger in or out until you see the center two circles on Row 1 overlap to form a cross.

5. Drop your finger but continue looking at that point in space where your finger was. You will know that you are doing this when you continue to see the fused image of the cross in the background.

6. Hold for 20 seconds.

7. Close your eyes and rest for 15 - 20 seconds.

8. Repeat again with the same row.

9. Repeat steps 5 - 8 with each of the three other rows.

What to watch for

1. You will probably find that either part 1 or part 2 is harder to do. For most benefit, practice the part that is harder.

2. For best results, follow this practice session with 5 - 10 minutes of Palming (P. 78) or any of the visualizations in this book.

3. Breathe steadily and naturally, relax your body and blink regularly. Look in a relaxed and easy way. Do not force or strain your eyes to see.

4. If the fused image fades out, briefly close your eyes, take a deep breath and relax. Then re-open your eyes and continue.

5. It is normal to find it easier to fuse certain rows. The value of using the Peripheral and Fusion Chart comes from making the attempt to gain fusion. Your fusion ability will improve over time.

6. Create the fused image only on the row that you are regarding. As you fuse this row, the other three will probably not be fused.

6. Peripheral Awareness Exercises

Purpose

To expand the range of your peripheral awareness and develop greater relaxation while concentrating.

6A. Pencil Awareness

REPETITIONS 5 times

TIME 10 minutes

MATERIALS Two pencils

SET UP

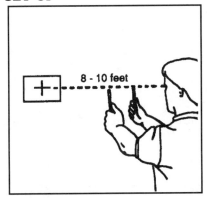

Fig. 23A Set up for PENCIL AWARENESS by standing 8-10 feet from a wall target, holding a pencil in each hand.

1. Stand directly in front of a target (a clock, calendar, etc.) that is at eye height on a wall 8 - 10 feet away. Hold a pencil in each hand in front of each eye. (Fig. 23A)

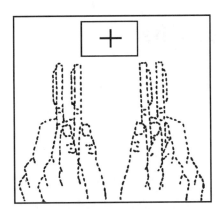 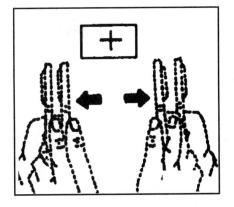

Fig. 23B When focused on the wall target, you'll see four images of the pencil in the foreground. Move the pencils apart while maintaining the four images (Fig. 23C).

Instructions

1. Focus on the wall target. In the foreground, see two images of each pencil. Blink and breathe. (Fig. 23B)

2. Keeping focused on the wall target, gradually move the pencils to the sides of your vision. Maintain your awareness of the four images until the pencils are too far apart to see the four images. Then, move the pencils in random directions — in and out, back and forth — keeping your focus on the wall target and maintaining your awareness of the four images of the pencils. Do this for 1 minute. (Fig. 23C)

3. Palm (P. 78) for 1 minute.

4. Repeat steps 1 - 2 four more times.

What to watch for

1. If you lose awareness of the double images, close your eyes, take a deep breath, then reopen your eyes and continue.

2. Remember to blink lightly and often, to keep your body relaxed, and to breathe regularly and easily.

3. It is helpful to have color contrast between the pencils and the wall target (i.e., dark pencils and light background) and the target should have good contrast against the wall as well.

6B. Peripheral Awareness Chart

REPETITIONS 10 times
TIME 10 minutes
MATERIALS NEEDED Peripheral Awareness Chart (P. 185)

SET UP

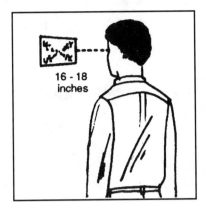

Fig. 24A   Stand 8-10 feet away from the Peripheral Awareness Chart, making sure that the center of the chart is at eye level.

1. Attach the Peripheral Awareness Chart to the wall at eye level and stand 16 - 18 inches from the chart. (Fig. 24A)

Instructions

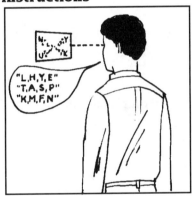

Fig. 24B   Focus on the letter in the center of the chart and call out all the other letters that you can read, without moving your eyes.

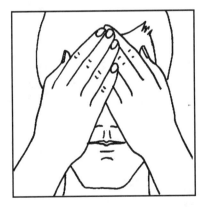

Fig. 24C   When finished, PALM to relax your eyes and mind.

1. Focus on the letter in the center of the chart. Without moving your eyes, call out the letters on the first ring. Continue looking at the center letter as you call out the letters in each successive ring. Blink and breathe and be aware of your periphery. (Fig. 24B)

2. When you have read as many letters as you can, close your eyes and palm over both eyes. Relax your brow as you take 3 deep breaths. (Fig. 24C)

3. Repeat four more times.

What to watch for

1. Through the repetition of regular and consistent practice you will be able to call out all the letters on the chart as you stay focused on the letter in the center.

2. As your peripheral awareness expands, you will notice certain letters on the chart become clearer and sharper as you remain focused on the center letter.

3. Make sure that you are standing correctly and keep your head straight and not tilted or turned.

4. You may find it helpful, before calling out letters, to increase your mental awareness of your peripheral vision, i.e., the edges of the card.

7. Unlocking Your Memory

Purpose

To unlock the part of your mind that stores your memories and to re-awaken your innate ability to remember, imagine and see.

REPETITIONS --

TIME 15 - 20 minutes

Instructions

1. Sit in a comfortable position and close your eyes, take a few full, deep breaths and relax.

2. Open your eyes and write the phrase, *"An early memory I have is ..."* on your paper.

3. Complete the phrase with whatever early memory comes to mind.

4. Write the phrase *"An early memory I have is ..."* again and complete it with another memory.

5. Continue writing and completing the phrase for 15 - 20 minutes, each time completing it with a different memory.

What to watch for

1. It is not necessary to write a detailed description of the memory. The purpose of the exercise is to awaken the visual memories in your mind, not to record every detail on paper. For example, writing *"an early memory I have is going fishing with my father"* is sufficient — as it crosses your mind and you write it down, the visual mind is reawakened. (You don't need to write down all the details of the fishing expedition!)

2. Be completely honest. Do not censor anything thoughts or memories; write them down without censoring.

3. If your mind goes blank, repeating out loud the phrase *"an early memory I have is ..."* 3 or 4 times should re-stimulate your awareness.

4. Don't force yourself to focus on any particular period of your life, but do lead yourself further and further back in time. Writing down things that happened yesterday or last week is not going to be as valuable as recalling events that occurred years ago.

Variations

1. Instead of writing, do this exercise out loud, looking at yourself in the mirror. For maximum value, do not hesitate or pause. If your mind goes blank, just keep saying out loud the phrase *"an early memory I have is ..."* again and again until a memory surfaces.

2. Do this exercise (either written or in the mirror) thinking particularly about your **Transitional Period** — that period of time 1 - 3 years before you first noticed a problem with your vision. (P. 44 - 48)

8. Vision Rock

Purpose

1. To stretch the focal range of your vision.

REPETITIONS 2 times (with each eye)
TIME 20 minutes
MATERIALS NEEDED   Dot Chart (P. 187)

                                         Eye patch (optional)

Instructions

1. Cover one eye with your hand (or an eye patch) and keep the covered eye open.

2. Hold the Dot Chart in front of the open eye. If you are nearsighted, hold the chart just *beyond* the distance at which you can see the top dot clearly. If you can still see the top dot clearly at arm's length, use a smaller dot. If you are farsighted, hold the chart just *closer* to you than the distance at which you can see the top dot clearly.

3. Keep your focus on the dot and with a slow, steady motion, move the chart closer to you until it is 2 - 3 inches from your eye.

4. Continue to keep your focus on the dot as you slowly move the chart away, until your arm is outstretched.

5. Continue moving the chart in and out as you stay focused on the dot. Continue for 3 - 4 minutes.

6. Palm (P. 78) over both closed eyes for 1 minute.

7. Repeat steps 2 - 6 again; if you can, focus on a smaller dot.

8. Palm over both closed eyes for 1 minute.

9. Repeat steps 2 - 8 with the other eye.

What to watch for

1. Move the chart slowly.

1. At some distances, the dot will be out of focus, but you may notice that you can keep it in focus within a greater and greater range as you continue to practice.

2. As you progress, focus on a smaller dot.

3. Do not try or strain to see more clearly. Relax your eyes and your focusing. Accept what you are seeing, even if it changes from moment to moment.

4. Relax any subtle tension that you might experience in your eyes, your jaw or the back of your neck.

5. Remember to breathe regularly. Blink once every 3 - 5 seconds.

6. The dot may go in and out of focus. That is a good sign.

9. Visual And Muscular Flexibility

Purpose

1. To regain greater flexibility and tone in the extra-ocular muscles, ciliary muscles and ciliary body.

2. To develop greater mind/eye coordination and balance.

REPETITIONS   4 sets (one eye at a time)

                    4 more sets (with both eyes)

TIME   30 - 35 minutes

MATERIALS NEEDED   I Love To See Chart (P. 189)

                        Metronome

                        Visual and Muscular Flexibility Audiotape (optional)

                        Eye Patch (optional)

SET UP

1. Place the I Love To See Chart on the wall so that the center of the chart is at eye level. You can do this technique either sitting or standing.

2. Sit (or stand) 8 - 10 feet from the chart.

Instructions (1 eye at a time)

1. Cover your right eye with an eye patch. Keep the covered eye open.

2. Pick a letter on the chart as your distant focus point. Hold your index finger 6 - 8 inches directly in front of your left eye and slightly below the letter. (Then, when you shift your focus in and out between the letter to your finger, your eyes will not move from right to left.)

3. Set the metronome at 30 beats per minute. Shift your focus from your finger to the letter in time with the beats, making one shift per beat.

4. Continue for 3 minutes.

5. Palm (P. 78) over both closed eyes for 1 - 2 minutes.

6. Repeat steps 3 - 5 with the metronome set to 45 beats per minute.

7. Repeat steps 3 - 5 with the metronome set to 60 beats per minute.

8. Repeat steps 3 - 5 with the metronome set to 72 beats per minute.

Instructions (both eyes):

1. Hold your index finger 6 - 8 inches directly in front of your nose with the letter on the chart behind your finger.

2. Repeat steps 3 - 8 above.

What to watch for

1. Even at the fastest speeds of the metronome, there is always enough time for your eyes to shift focus in and out if you and your eyes are relaxed and fluid. It is a sign of excessive visual control if it doesn't feel that way. Try to gain the feeling that your eyes are moving by themselves, rather than you moving them. Allow your eye movements to become as relaxed, effortless and fluid as possible.

2. Make sure that your focus goes all the way to each target and rests on it briefly before you shift your vision to the other target.

3. Sense the difference in your visual system and eyes as you focus on the near and far targets. As you continue to practice, you will notice that the target you are directly looking at is seen more clearly than the other.

4. Remember to breathe steadily, blink regularly and stay relaxed.

Variation

Use the Fusion String (P. 64) instead of your finger and the chart. With one eye covered with an eye patch, hold the Fusion String directly in front of the open eye; with both eyes, hold the Fusion String to the tip of your nose. *If you are nearsighted,* make the near target the farthest bead that you can see with clarity and the distant target the first or second bead *beyond* your range of clarity. As you improve, use a farther bead as the distant target and a closer bead as the near target. *If you are farsighted,* make bead 6 the distant target. Make the near target the farthest bead from your eyes that is not clear. As you improve, use a closer bead at near and a farther bead at far.

PART 5:

WHAT ELSE YOU NEED TO KNOW

CHAPTER NINETEEN

HOW TO MONITOR YOUR PROGRESS

"In order to see more clearly, I have to take notice of what I can already see, rather than look for what I should be able to see but can't."
—I Touch The Earth, The Earth Touches Me, Hugh Prather

"I See"

It is important to acknowledge yourself for all the progress you are making. Whether the improvement is small or large, lasts for a fraction of a second or an hour, every time that you notice a positive change in your vision — whether it's during a practice session or at any other time of the day — say to yourself the acknowledging phrase, "I SEE." You will be surprised at the response that this affirmation builds inside of you.

Changes to look for

As your vision improves it will go through many stages of change. Some of these stages will be obvious signs of improvement while others will be periods of readjustment marked by the surfacing and releasing of old, long-held patterns of emotional stress and physical tension.

Here are the most common signs of improvement. (You may or may not experience all of them.)

Physical signs

- More energy and vitality
- Blurriness becoming more distinct
- Black appearing blacker (and, at first, not necessarily clearer)
- Colors looking brighter and more vivid
- Greater clarity and a sense of the three-dimensionality of things
- Eyes more opened and relaxed; feeling less tense

- Less sensitivity to sunlight (less of a need to use sunglasses)
- Brief moments of improved vision
- Body more relaxed
- Better depth perception
- Greater peripheral awareness

Mental signs

- More vivid recall of dreams
- Increased imagination and creative expression
- Better and clearer memory
- More natural tendency toward positive thinking
- Sharper mental focus
- Greater power of concentration
- Greater ability to see tasks all the way through to the end

Emotional signs

- Greater self acceptance
- Greater self esteem
- More self confidence
- More emotional dreams
- Increased sense of connectedness to self and to others
- Greater sensitivity to self and to others
- More desire to express loving, caring and compassion
- Greater acceptance of the past and of its useful value
- More acceptance and resolve with emotionally disturbing issues
- Greater self honesty
- Deeper willingness to see things for what they are

Readjustment periods

None of the techniques in this book can put tension or stress into your eyes or your body. However, they can help to surface deeply ingrained physical and emotional tension. These periods of release and readjustment often precede changes in physical eyesight. Though these periods may be temporarily uncomfortable, knowing what to expect if and when you should experience them will make it easier for you to let the old patterns of physical tension and emotional stress run their natural course as they leave your body.

Possible symptoms of readjustment

- Headaches
- Temporary aches in your shoulders, neck and throat
- Eyes feeling "worked out"
- Tingling or vibrating in the back of your head and neck
- Tearing, watering, stinging or burning of your eyes
- Twitching spasms in your eyelids or around your eyes
- Increased discharge ("sleepdust") from your eyes
- Temporary periods of double vision
- Changes in your sense of balance or in orientation
- Greater awareness of your emotions
- Awareness of your changing attitudes

An effective way to move through these readjustment periods as quickly as possible is to work actively with the weekly positive thoughts or with any of the Vision Affirmations (P. 169).

If you are uncertain about any readjustment symptoms that you are experiencing, contact The Cambridge Institute (508-887-3883) for assistance, clarification and guidance.

CHAPTER TWENTY

10 HABITS FOR BETTER VISION

Since you use your eyes during most of your waking hours, incorporating proper visual habits into your awareness can go a long way towards keeping your eyes stress free and helping your visual system. It requires no extra time. All it takes is the awareness of how to use your eyes and mind.

Some of the 10 visual habits will keep your eyes working in a relaxed, normal way, preventing you from accumulating visual stress. Others will make you more mentally alert and focused and encourage you to become more emotionally involved in what you are seeing and feeling.

Make these habits second nature and you'll soon start to experience the benefits.

1. Blink regularly: Blinking cleanses and lubricates the eyes. When there is no tension, your eyes blink 10 - 12 times every minute, or about once every 5 seconds. But people who do not see clearly tend to unconsciously stare and hold their eyes open, which causes strain as well as the feeling of dry and tired eyes.

Consciously remind yourself to blink every 3 - 5 seconds. Of course, you don't want to go through the day with a stopwatch, but the more conscious you are of blinking regularly, the better it is for your eyes.

The eyelid is the only part of the body that is controlled by just one muscle. By having proper tone and relaxation in that muscle, it can promote relaxation throughout the entire body. (That's why a hypnotist often uses the phrase *"your eyes are becoming heavy"* as a way to get the subject to become more relaxed.)

Flutter Blinking is one exercise that you can use any time during the day when you catch yourself staring or when your eyes feel strained or tired. To practice **Flutter Blinking**, blink your eyes lightly and rapidly 10 - 20 times. Do not strain or squeeze your eyes shut; instead, relax your face as you blink. Then close your eyes for a moment and relax. Repeat this 2 or 3 times. **Flutter Blinking** will help to keep your eyes moist, relaxed and free of strain.

2. Use Your Peripheral Vision: At the same time that you are focusing on an object, images are also coming into your eyes from your peripheral awareness — from the sides and from in front of and behind what you are directly looking at. Relaxed and balanced vision requires the organized and coordinated use of both your central and peripheral vision.

People with poor vision often lock their concentration so intently on just one thing that they block out their peripheral awareness. This "putting on blinders" breeds mental fatigue and a tense style of concentration.

Always strive to be aware of your total field of vision — the desk that the book you are reading is on, the space between you and the vision chart, or your surroundings as you drive down the road, for example.

3. Keep your eyes moving and change your focus: Staring is the most commonly practiced bad habit by people who do not see clearly. Keeping your eyes moving and changing your focus is the most direct and powerful way to break the staring habit.

The eyes are in constant motion, scanning the environment so often and moving so rapidly that they send 60 - 70 images to the mind **every second**! This steady, subtle movement is essential for clear vision; staring and freezing your eye movements interferes with the normal functioning of the visual system.

Of course, you can't consciously move your eyes that fast, but you can unlock tension in your visual system by remembering to change your focus frequently.

This encourages your eyes to become more relaxed.

Whatever you are looking at, remember to shift your focus and keep your eyes moving. For example, when driving a car, shift your focus from the speedometer to the rear view mirror to the license plate of the car in front of you, and so on. Whether walking down the street, watching TV or engaged in conversation, you can always keep your eyes moving and change your focus regularly.

When reading or doing other close work such as using a computer, it is especially important that you look up and focus on something in the distance at least once every 2 - 3 minutes.

A powerful vision-improving combination is to expand your peripheral awareness while you are moving your eyes and shifting your focus.

4. Avoid daydreaming: You can tell when somebody is daydreaming: they get a glazed, de-focused look in their eyes, they stare, they don't blink and their eyes don't move. All of which, when it becomes a habit, promotes poor vision.

In this context, daydreaming means any mental activity — whether or not it involves images — that captures a person's inner focus while their eyes are open.

Stay present and aware. Being involved in the present moment assists you in keeping your mental focus and physical eyesight working together.

There isn't anything wrong with the creative use of the imagination, but when daydreaming becomes a habit it can have a negative effect on your vision.

Here's why:

If you close your eyes and imagine looking at a distant scene, your eyes respond to that, and change their focus, as they would if they were actually looking at that distant scene. It is as if your physical eyes are trying to focus on what you see in your mind's eye.

So, if you're driving down the road and you're thinking about something else, your eyes are caught in a dilemma — what should they be seeing? On the one hand, they are trying to bring the road into focus and on the other hand, they are trying to focus on what's in your mind. This causes you to stare, creates visual tension and sends mixed messages to the visual centers of the brain.

Don't let your eyes get stuck between these two different kinds of seeing — the outer sight and the inner vision. Close your eyes when you want to daydream. And stay involved in your world when your eyes are open.

The need for glasses increases as students go further along in school. What are most of these kids doing in school? Most of the time, they're daydreaming about what they're going to do *after* school — while their eyes are trying to focus on the blackboard.

But there is another "daydream" that students are involved in every single day: Reading. When reading, the eyes are seeing the letters on the page (for example they might be seeing the letters C A T). But in your mind you see the image of a cat. Your eyes are seeing one thing and your mind is seeing another.

Sustained focusing at near has been cited as a major cause of nearsightedness, but reading — because it is an abstract activity — can be particularly stressful to the eyes.

To prevent reading from stressing the eyes, make sure that you practice habits 1 - 3 when you read.

It's just as important to remember to be conscious of what you are actually seeing — the letters on the page — as well as being absorbed in what the words mean to you.

Teach these tips to your children, too! And help them maintain and protect the vision that they were born with.

5. Look with the "eyes of a child": If you are diligently remembering to blink, to move your eyes, shift focus, to use your peripheral vision and to avoid daydreaming, you could get stuck in the trap of using your eyes in a mechanical way.

There's a big difference between passively seeing and actively looking. There's always something new and different to notice. Engage your visual world as a child would — with excitement, awe and wonder — as if everything you are seeing is new and fresh.

6. Nourish and rest your eyes: Natural sunlight is a nutrient for the body just like food and water. The eyes see best in natural light. The fact that most of us spend nearly all day under artificial light has far-reaching consequences for our vision and our overall health.

To get the light nourishment that your eyes and body need, spend *at least* 30 minutes a day outdoors — without glasses or contacts — so that your visual system can receive unfiltered sunlight. Any glass — window glass, car windshield, eyeglasses or contacts — filters part of the full spectrum of light and reduces the beneficial effect that sunlight has on your eyes and body. We recommend sunglasses in situations of glare or reflected light (the beach or ski slopes). The sunglasses we do recommend are "neutral gray." That is, they filter all parts of the light spectrum equally. (Contact The Cambridge Institute for information.)

Recently, there has been some concern about the depletion of the protective ozone layer and the potentially harmful effects of too much sunlight. There is some indication that it is not the exposure to sunlight that is harmful, but rather exposure only after a prolonged lack of exposure (*i.e.,* spending day after day indoors under artificial light). Though it might be wise to limit sunbathing and other extreme exposure to sunlight, it is still very important for the health of your eyes (and your body) to be exposed to natural sunlight on a regular basis for at least some time each day.

The kind of indoor lighting that you use is also important. Dr. John Ott, a pioneer in the field of photobiology (the study of how different kinds of light affect living organisms), developed an indoor light that is the most complete substitute for sunlight. It is called Vita-Lite and it easily replaces any standard fluorescent tube. Studies have shown that using Vita-Lite increases see-ability, reduces glare and eyestrain and improves visual acuity.

Your eyes most fully rest in total darkness. The best way to rest your eyes is to close them and place your cupped palms over your closed eyes (see Palming, P. 78). You can palm for as little as 30 - 40 seconds any time that your eyes feel tired or strained. While palming, it is also helpful to visualize a pleasant scene in your mind's eye.

Nourishing and resting your eyes is best accomplished at the same time by doing the **Sun Cycle**:

The Sun Cycle

1. *Close* your eyes and face toward the sun. (If you cannot face the sun with your eyes closed without squinting or tightening your facial muscles, then begin the **Sun Cycle** by facing slightly away from the sun so that your face and closed eyes can relax. Then, as you become more accustomed to the light, gradually turn closer and closer towards the sun.)

2. Let the sunlight fall on your closed eyes for five seconds.

3. Palm over your closed eyes, shutting out all light for five more seconds, then take your hands away, keeping your eyes **closed**.

4. Repeat steps 1 - 3 ten to twenty times, for a total of three to five minutes.

The **Sun Cycle** helps to nourish your visual system, exercise the focusing muscles of the eyes and reduce sensitivity to glare.

In most cases people who are overly sensitive to natural sunlight have starved their visual systems of this important nutrient. It is especially beneficial for them to practice the **Sun Cycle**; they should begin to experience a decrease in sensitivity within twenty to thirty days.

7. Use an under-corrected prescription: If you wear glasses or contacts, you have probably experienced the all too familiar pattern of needing a stronger and stronger prescription year after year. A number of factors contribute to this decline, but to a large degree this decline can be prevented by using an under-corrected prescription.

If you are nearsighted and use an under-corrected prescription, you probably won't be able to read the bottom line on the eye chart. You could read one or two lines above the bottom line, yet this under-corrected prescription would be strong enough for you to drive safely.(and legally) and to see comfortably in almost every situation. If you use reading glasses, you might need to hold the reading material a little farther than normal from your eyes in order to read it.

An under-corrected prescription encourages your visual system to work with the glasses or contacts — and not just passively depend on them — in order to see. If you are also doing eye exercises, then as your vision improves what was once an under-corrected prescription will eventually become too strong as your own vision gets clearer. Then, you would be ready for another, even weaker, under-corrected prescription.

In this way you are slowly weaning yourself from corrective lenses and your eyesight gets stronger as your glasses or contacts get weaker. (See **Visiting The Eye Doctor**, Pp. 54 - 56.)

8. Increase body relaxation and good posture: Postural imbalances and physical tension have long been associated with vision problems, so it's important for you to find ways to release tension and develop relaxation in your body.

Your vision is affected by tension in your body, particularly in the upper part — the chest, shoulders, neck and face. Remember to relax your forehead and shoulders and "loosen" your jaw. This encourages the oxygen and blood supply to move freely and easily through your entire visual system.

Additionally, any cleansing of the body — particularly the circulatory and lymphatic systems — will help clear away toxins that may inhibit clear vision.

9. Breathe deeply and regularly: Approximately 30% of the oxygen you inhale goes to nourish the muscles, nerves and brain cells of your visual system.

Watch what happens the next time you are tense or engrossed in an activity. Most likely your breathing will become shallow and irregular. You might even find that you are unconsciously holding your breath some of the time.

Breathe deeply and rhythmically. It helps vision. And it will keep your body more relaxed, help you concentrate easier for longer periods of time and eliminate eyestrain and fatigue.

Any aerobic physical activity (swimming, running, brisk walking, etc.) assists in improving your vision. Perform these activities without glasses or contacts whenever possible.

10. Look openly and honestly: Past and present emotional stress and resistance to facing what you see can affect vision. It is important to develop the inner willingness to see.

Emotionally, there may be a part of us that believes that if we don't see something it might disappear. Though this response might make us feel more safe, nothing disappears when we don't see it. Instead, the problem or the feeling haunts us until we look at it and deal with it openly and directly.

Develop a deeper willingness to look honestly and openly at challenging and difficult situations. Look for the positive potential in all situations. This is particularly helpful when things aren't going your way!

Consciously develop these 10 habits until they become second nature and your eyes and body will start to feel more relaxed and your seeing will become clearer. You will start to develop a whole new way of looking and perceiving that involves your eyes, your mind and your heart.

CHAPTER TWENTY ONE

TECHNIQUES YOU CAN DO THROUGHOUT THE DAY

There are many techniques that you can practice during spare moments throughout the day. In fact, some people get quite creative — setting up a Fusion String by the telephone or even placing a vision chart at the office.

Use your imagination and you'll be surprised by how many different ways you can incorporate these techniques into your life. Your eyes will be glad that you did!

Here are some suggestions for good things you can do for your eyes throughout each and every day.

If you have one minute or less:
Eye Stretches (Pp. 84 - 86)
Eye Squeezes (Pp. 88 - 89)
Five-Finger Eye Massage (Pp. 73 - 74)
Three-Finger Eye Massage (Pp. 74 - 75
Energy Transfer Point Massage (Pp. 75 - 76)

If you have two to five minutes:
Fusion String (Pp. 64 - 68)
The Sun Cycle (Pp. 163)
Palming (P. 78)
Swinging (Pp. 69 - 71)

You can always do:
Near-To-Far Shifting (Pp. 81 - 82)
Corner-To-Corner Shifting (Pp. 83 - 84)
Repeating Vision Affirmations (Pp. 167 - 169)

CHAPTER TWENTY TWO

USING AFFIRMATIONS FOR BETTER VISION

Another way to clarify self image and perspective and to release unconscious limiting thoughts and beliefs is to use the principle of affirmations, which are vision-promoting thoughts.

Subtle patterns and attitudes become implanted in your subconscious over time and although you may no longer consciously remember what is hidden inside, it still influences how you see, both literally and figuratively. Affirmations are an excellent way to surface, release and let go of deeply rooted beliefs that may still be unconsciously limiting your vision.

The value of developing a positive attitude is to learn to accept what you see and to consciously fill your mind with thoughts that focus directly on what you want to create and experience.

For example, it may seem "true" to say *"I can't see,"* but that thought only reinforces the existing limitation. Saying, *"I am looking to notice what I can see,"* reinforces the opposite — the desire to have clearer vision.

Over the years, at one time or another, the list of negative and critical thoughts about your vision may have included these statements:

1. "My eyes are bad."
2. "My eyes are weak."
3. "I inherited poor vision."
4. "I can't see."
5. "I'm under a lot of stress."
6. "My job ruined my eyes."
7. "I'll never be able to see any better."

8. "If I don't wear my glasses my eyes will get worse."

9. "I've been wearing glasses too long to give them up."

10. "What I don't see won't hurt me."

Here's one way to change these negative statements into affirmations:

1. My eyes are beautiful.

2. My eyes have all the power and strength they need to see clearly.

3. God created me with perfect vision.

4. I am seeing more clearly every day.

5. I am handling life's challenges successfully without strain or effort.

6. I can change my vision if I want to.

7. My vision is changing for the better all the time.

8. I have the power to change my vision.

9. I can regain clear vision regardless of my age.

10. The more I see, the safer I feel.

Affirmation Writing Exercise

Select an affirmation from one of the eight weekly positive thoughts in THE FIRST STAGE schedule, from the list that follows or, if you wish, make up your own.

Then, take a piece of paper, draw a line down the center, and at the top of the left side of the page write, "Affirmation," and on the right, "Response."

Now, in the "Affirmation" column, write the affirmation you selected and record your first reaction to it in the "Response" column. Whether it be a thought, a feeling or a physical reaction write it down. Then write the affirmation again and record your reaction again. For example:

Affirmation	Response
I am seeing clearly.	But I still see things blurred.
I am seeing clearly.	I can't let go.
I am seeing clearly.	Tears.

Continue doing this for 15 minutes, recording your honest responses. Don't censor them no matter how silly, judgmental or "off-the-wall" they seem to be. Your responses may be in opposition to the affirmation. That's okay. Just write them down. When the 15 minutes are up, close your eyes and take a few more minutes to reflect on the affirmation.

Affirmation Writing is an excellent exercise to do in the morning before you begin your day or late at night before you go to bed. During the day you can also repeat the affirmation to yourself every time you remember it. You might even want to carry the affirmation on a card in your wallet or put the card up on your bathroom mirror or have a copy of it on your desk at work.

List of Affirmations

1. My eyes are beautiful.
2. I am pleased with the way I see.
3. My eyes are a safe and pleasurable place for me.
4. It is easy for me to see clearly.
5. I am safe even when my vision is unclear.
6. I love to relax.
7. The more ease and relaxation I allow myself, the clearer I see.
8. The more I relax, the more I accomplish.
9. There is always enough time for me to see anything that I choose clearly.
10. The muscles in and around my eyes are moving freely and easily.
11. I can see clearly with or without my glasses.
12. My body, mind and emotions cooperate in clearing my vision.
13. My memory and imagination serve me perfectly.
14. My clear memory of difficult situations is allowing me to balance my emotions with love.
15. I can imagine anything I want clearly.
16. I am letting go of anything between me and my goal of clear vision.
17. I accept the gift of clear vision.
18. I am giving the gifts of aliveness and clarity to myself and others.
19. I am now seeing all the beauty and love in and around me.
20. I forgive myself for thinking I hated anyone.
21. I forgive others for thinking they hated me.
22. As my heart opens, my vision clears.

Changing your limiting thoughts and beliefs about your vision is an integral part of gaining **Better Vision**. Using affirmations can greatly assist you to make changes in both your vision and your life.

CHAPTER TWENTY THREE

ADVICE FOR SPECIFIC PROBLEMS

Nearsightedness, farsightedness, astigmatism and eye imbalance are functional vision problems. They are the result of how the brain and the eyes function together. On the surface they may seem to be different problems, but the same underlying factors addressed in this book contribute to each of them.

As you correct these underlying factors the different parts of your visual system will be brought into greater balance and your specific problems will diminish and can eventually disappear.

That's why it is necessary for each person — regardless of the specific problem(s) involved — to practice the same First Stage Eight Week Schedule (Pp. 106 - 121). This schedule brings to your awareness the underlying difficulties affecting your vision. By practicing the First Stage you'll start to release the tension and stress affecting your visual system, train the eyes and brain to work better together and change the inner issues affecting vision.

Only after completing the First Stage Eight Week Schedule should you address your specific problem(s) by using the techniques listed below. Don't make the mistake of skipping the First Stage; you'll do your vision a disservice because you won't be laying the proper foundation for improvement.

Sharpening emotional clarity, releasing inner blocks to seeing and enhancing concentration and mental focus are always important — and will greatly aid improvement for all the functional vision problems. You may find that at different times in your process you'll gain more benefit from some visualizations than you will at other times. Experiment and be flexible in your approach.

Also, consider using the nutritional supplements listed on P. 201; they are helpful for all functional vision problems.

(Techniques are listed in alphabetical order , not in order of importance.)

Releasing inner blocks and sharpening emotional clarity:
    Affirmation Writing (Pp. 167 - 169)
    Developing the Inner Seer (Pp. 132)
    Forgiveness (P. 199 - 200)
    Memory Visualization (Pp. 97 - 101)
    Unlocking Your Memory (Pp. 147 - 148)

Enhancing concentration and mental focus:
    Corner-to-Corner Shifting (Pp. 83 - 84)
    Edging (Pp. 86 - 88)
    Mind's Eye Visualization (Pp. 90 - 92)
    Spectrum Visualization (Pp. 93 - 96)

Nearsightedness (myopia):
    Exploring Your "Blur Zone" (Pp. 133 - 134)
    Fusion String Technique (one eye at a time) (variation 1) (P. 67)
    Letting Go of Visual Tension (Pp. 135 - 138)
    Peripheral Awareness Exercises (Pp. 143 - 146)
    Self Massage Techniques (Pp. 69 - 78)
    Vision Chart Techniques (Pp. 79 - 89)
    Visual and Muscular Flexibility (Pp. 151 - 152)

Farsightedness (hyperopia):
    Exploring Your "Blur Zone" (Pp. 133 - 134)
    Fusion String Technique (one eye at a time) (variation 2) (P. 67)
    Letting Go of Visual Tension (Pp. 135 - 138)
    Self Massage Techniques (Pp. 69 - 78)
    Vision Chart Techniques (Pp. 79 - 89)
    Vision Rock (Pp. 149 - 150)
    Visual and Muscular Flexibility (Pp. 151 - 152)

Astigmatism:

Energy Transfer Point (Pp. 75 - 76)

Eye Stretches (variation 1) (P. 85)

Eye Squeezes (Pp. 88 - 89)

Fusion String Technique (one eye at a time) (variation 3) (P. 67)

Head Rolls (Pp. 71 - 72)

Peripheral Awareness Exercises (Pp. 143 - 146)

Self Massage Techniques (Pp. 69 - 78)

Differences between the eyes:

Balance and Coordination Exercises (Pp. 128 - 131)

Energy Transfer Point (Pp. 75 - 76)

Fusion String Technique (Pp. 64 - 68)

Near-to-Far Shifting (Pp. 81 - 82)

Peripheral and Fusion Awareness (Pp. 139 - 142)

Self Massage Techniques (Pp. 69 - 78)

Spectrum Visualization (Pp. 93 - 96)

Visual and Muscular Flexibility (Pp. 151 - 152)

For personal advice for your situation, including new techniques and an individualized advanced schedule, contact Martin Sussman (508-887-3884) to find out how you can get a personal consultation.

CHAPTER TWENTY FOUR

SAVING YOUR EYES AT THE COMPUTER

NOTE: Many of these suggestions are beneficial to practice when engaged in any type of close range focus, i.e. reading, sewing, painting, etc.

Using a computer places a unique set of demands on the visual system. Without proper training and good visual habits, the eyes and body can suffer. It's not uncommon for computer users to experience eyestrain, vision headaches, deteriorating vision and the need for stronger and stronger prescriptions, as well as other uncomfortable and painful symptoms.

Altogether, there are seven keys to taking care of your eyes at the computer. The first three ensure that your work area promotes healthy visual habits:

1. Maximize focusing distance
2. Eliminate glare
3. Light the room appropriately

Achieving these three will help to create an environment in which you can optimally use and rest your eyes. It will also give you a head start on being able to eliminate two of the major sources of physical and mental fatigue — glare and eyestrain.

To keep your vision as clear and relaxed as it can be, practice and integrate the next four keys and use them while working at the computer:

4. Blink every 3 to 5 seconds
5. See more than the screen
6. Look into the distance frequently
7. Use computer glasses if appropriate

Correct blinking, "opening up" your vision (being aware of surroundings while looking at the screen), and taking short vision breaks will keep your eyes healthy and relaxed, your vision clear, and increase your ability to concentrate easily.

Let's look at each of these seven keys more closely.

1. Maximize focusing distance

Set your computer up in your workspace so that you can look beyond the screen to the farthest object in the room. Being able to look up into the distance is the most important way that you can rest your eyes during computer work. Rest prevents the accumulation of visual stress.

If possible, you *don't* want to be in the corner of the room or face a wall or window. Window light is another source of unwanted stress. Instead, try facing a doorway so your distance view is down the hall.

TIP: If your computer is in a corner or if you work in a small space, place a small mirror on top of your monitor or on your desk. Use the mirror to give your eyes a distant view by looking through the mirror and focusing on objects that you see behind you.

2. Eliminate glare

Glare is any light or image reflected off the VDT screen that reaches the eyes, cannot be ignored and competes for visual attention.

Sources of glare may be the lights in the room, the light fixtures themselves, unshaded windows, or bright objects, such as your own white shirt or blouse.

Glare silently forces you to (unconsciously) twist and turn your head and body to avoid it. And your eyes do have to work harder to focus on the information on the screen (which leads to eyestrain and strain of the neck, back, shoulders and arms).

You can tell there's reflected glare by turning on the lights in the room before turning on your computer. If you see any images or reflections on the (turned-off) screen, you've got a glare problem.

To reduce or minimize glare, experiment by:
* Tilting the screen
* Moving objects that reflect *onto* the screen
* Covering windows to block sunlight
* Turning off or lowering offending lights
* Covering fluorescent lights with egg-crate baffles
* Turning your computer so the screen is perpendicular to
overhead fluorescent lights.

This may do it. However, since most offices were not designed or built for computer work it may be impossible to eliminate glare altogether, in which case you might consider using an anti-glare screen.

Anti-glare screens

Adding an anti-glare screen to your monitor is a way to filter out unwanted glare, and a wise investment in your health and comfort. A good anti-glare screen also increases the contrast of characters against the background, making it easier for your eyes to see.

Low-quality screens should be avoided because they can cut down the resolution and clarity of the characters on the screen, which encourages eyestrain and fatigue.

Anti-glare sprays are available, but anti-glare screens are much more effective.

Another form of glare is light that originates from the computer screen itself. This happens when the brightness control is turned up too high and you are viewing dark letters against a bright background.

Tinted glasses

Many offices are over illuminated for computer work and often overhead lights cannot be turned off. If you cannot control ambient lighting it is worth discussing with a behavioral optometrist (see Pp. 54 - 56) whether or not you should use tinted glasses.

If your workstation is well laid out and you have good control of ambient lighting, most of the time a tint on your glasses won't be necessary.

For an amber screen, a light-blue or blue-gray tint on your glasses is recommended. For a green screen, a rose or light-pink tint. In some cases a coating to block ultraviolet light provides increased comfort; in others, a light-gray or brown tint helps reduce the effects of excessive illumination.

3. Light the room appropriately

If you've completely eliminated all sources of glare onto your screen, chances are your workspace is now pretty dark. This is a problem because you don't want to be working in a darkened room.

Make sure that you have some overhead, background or foreground lighting.

And make sure you don't have a light source anywhere in your line of sight when you're looking at the screen. This will distract your peripheral vision and cause mental fatigue.

You also need to light any original copy that you are working from. A desk lamp with an adjustable neck works well. Just make sure that this light doesn't distract you or spill onto your VDT screen.

Hard copy tip: Ideally, you want your copy on the same vertical plane as the screen. Working side to side is preferable to looking from the screen down to your copy and then back up to the screen again. Alternate moving the written material that you work from to the left and right of the screen during the day. The eye movements required to shift back and forth from left to right and from screen to copy help reduce visual stress and enhance your visual skills.

If you have some control over the overhead illumination, adjustable incandescent light, especially indirect light, is often the most comfortable. Standing lamps that direct light at the ceiling provide the best indirect light. If there is no dimmer available, a 3-way fixture is recommended so you can set the light at the most comfortable level.

Do fluorescent lights bother your eyes or reflect onto your screen? Most problems are caused by the *quantity* of the light (not by fluorescence itself). If possible, turn off every other fluorescent fixture and light your desk with a 100-watt bulb. Or replace all fluorescent lights with Vita-Lite, a special fluorescent tube which emits a different *quality* of light which simulates the full spectrum of natural sunlight more closely than any other artificial light. This makes it easier on your eyes to see. It may also be appropriate to reduce the quantity of light even if you use Vita-Lite. (For more information, contact the Cambridge Institute, 508-887-3883.)

4. Blink every 3 to 5 seconds

Blinking lubricates and cleanses the eyes, keeping them moist for clear vision and comfort. Blinking also helps relax the facial muscles and forehead, countering the tendency to furrow one's brow and create tension.

Many people do not blink regularly. Instead, while concentrating intently, especially when under pressure, they keep their eyes wide open — fixed — and blinking decreases. Decreased blinking often causes redness, burning and itching of the eyes, particularly for those who use contact lenses.

To blink correctly: Move only your eyelids — not your forehead, face or cheeks. Make sure you close your eyes all the way without effort and that both the upper and lower lids touch gently. Make sure that your brow is relaxed. Blink lightly once every 3 to 5 seconds.

5. See more than the screen

Keep your vision "open."

This means that while looking at the screen you are also aware of your surroundings — the desk, the walls, people passing by, etc. Being more fully aware of your peripheral vision can significantly reduce visual stress, physical fatigue and mental tiredness.

You can expand your peripheral vision when looking directly at something by reminding yourself to be aware of objects to your right and left.

Total visual awareness promotes visual, physical and mental relaxation and will help you see more easily and clearly.

A thin line separates "concentration with attention" from "concentration with tension." To prevent yourself from crossing over this line keep your breathing full and relaxed, blink regularly and lightly, and "open" your peripheral vision.

Surprisingly, using your total visual awareness will help you focus more easily on what you are doing (concentration with attention) while at the same time prevent you from expending too much mental effort (concentration with tension).

6. Look into the distance frequently

Extended staring at a computer screen inevitably creates fatigue, tension and eye problems. Failing to take short vision breaks is one of the major factors leading to nearsightedness among computer users. Don't wait for your eyes to start hurting or for your vision to get blurry before taking short vision breaks on a regular basis.

Simple as it seems, a brief look into the distance every 2 to 3 minutes prevents the build-up of visual stress and discomfort and keeps your eyes healthy and active.

And, contrary to conventional wisdom, a break every hour — however long it might be — does not provide all the relief and rest that your eyes need. But a short vision break is effective and beneficial. Actually, this short break takes less time than a 5-minute break every hour.

Taking short vision breaks doesn't require "real" time, only "real" awareness, an awareness that you can develop.

Short vision break tip: Look up and focus on the furthest object in the distance. Be aware of objects around you in your periphery. Take a deep breath. Relax on the exhale. Blink correctly a couple of times. Shift your vision back to the screen and re-focus. (Three near-to-far shifts per break are recommended. This should take about 5 seconds.)

Short vision breaks will keep your eye muscles relaxed and flexible and prevent the accumulation of visual stress and fatigue. They'll also increase your ability to maintain concentration for longer periods of time as well as increase your accuracy and productivity over that period of time.

7. Use computer glasses if appropriate

All eyeglasses and contact lenses are not the same.

Whether or not you currently use either, you could benefit from using special "computer glasses." These "computer glasses" help relieve visual strain and halt the deterioration of vision that can sometimes accompany using a computer.

In fact, even if you do not presently need regular glasses or contacts, you can benefit from using "computer glasses" because they can help you maintain the good vision you already have.

What kind of special "computer glasses" you need depends on your particular vision problem.

(In addition to using "computer glasses," applying the principles in this book will help improve your ability to function more efficiently and effectively at the computer. If you presently need glasses/contacts, the correct and consistent application of these principles can initially lead to a reduction in the strength of your prescription and eventually to a reduced need to use them.)

If you use glasses/contacts for distance vision

Most people who use glasses for distance seeing are nearsighted and without their glasses near objects are clearer than distant ones. In fact, many nearsighted people see reasonably well close-up without glasses altogether.

However, when distance glasses are used for extended near work the result is often stress, fatigue, tension and reduced performance. Why? Because your eyes have to work even harder to bring the screen (a near object) into focus when you are using glasses that are supposed to help you focus in the distance. Over time, this leads to poorer vision and the need for stronger distance glasses.

Properly prescribed "computer glasses" for near seeing can provide relief from the stress of extended close work.

"Computer glasses" reduce stress on the focusing muscles of the eyes by making screen characters appear to the eyes a little larger and a little farther away.

If you use glasses/contacts for near vision

If you already use glasses for reading it does not necessarily mean that these are the ones you should be using for computer work. Near vision glasses are usually prescribed for about 16 inches viewing distance, but this may or may not be best for your particular computer situation.

If you are using bifocals you may find that the reading portion of the glasses is too low for the greatest ease of screen viewing. Your bifocals may also require you to make slight but uncomfortable adjustments of your neck (or back) to see the screen, this only adds to physical stress and discomfort by creating physical and mental fatigue.

It is often best to have a different prescription or a different type of lens for your computer work.

A single-vision glass set for computer distance, or a special bifocal, trifocal or "no-line bifocal" also may be appropriate.

If you do not use any glasses/contacts

If you use a computer, but do not use glasses or contacts, you still might be experiencing some kind of visual problem(s) that led you to read this book.

Even though you do not need regular everyday glasses, "computer glasses" might enhance your performance and/or help you maintain the good vision that you already have.

This is definitely worth looking into if you are experiencing any kind of visual or physical problems at all during computer work.

Contact a behavioral optometrist (Pp. 54 - 56) for assistance in getting "computer glasses."

This chapter is adapted from information that first appeared in the book, **Total Health at the Computer,** by Martin Sussman and Dr. Ernest Loewenstein with Howard Sann. Published by Station Hill Press. For information contact 508-887-3883.

PART 6:

APPENDIX

GLOSSARY OF TERMS

ACCOMMODATION — the ability of the eye to shift focus and have clear vision with ease.

ACUITY — the ability to see clearly.

BEHAVIORAL OPTOMETRIST — a specialist who evaluates vision not only in relation to clarity of sight, but who also takes into consideration efficiency and comfort, performance, posture and behavior. One goal (accomplished through vision training) is to restore and enhance visual abilities so that there is less need for glasses or contact lenses.

BLUR ZONE — the part of your visual world that is not in clear focus. There is an imaginary boundary line between the blur zone and the clear zone. The initial goal of vision improvement is to expand the range of the clear zone by regularly looking into the blur zone without glasses.

CENTRAL FIXATION/PERIPHERAL BALANCE — the balance between central fixation (the ability to see one point clearly) and the periphery (everything else in your total field of vision). Signs of poor peripheral awareness include a sense of insecurity when driving a car and bumping into objects or doorways when walking.

CILIARY MUSCLES — the muscles encircling the lens of your eyes which control the shape of the lens as it changes focus. These muscles are also involved in the functioning of the iris.

CONVERGENCE/BINOCULARITY — the balanced, coordinated teamwork of your eyes and brain that allows you to make accurate judgments in depth and distance. Signs of poor convergence include strain when reading for prolonged periods, difficulty maintaining concentration, under-developed eye/hand coordination, poor judgment of distances and susceptibility to tension headaches.

CROSS EYE/strabismus — the condition that exists when the brain does not use both eyes in a coordinated way.

FARSIGHTEDNESS/hyperopia — the difficulty of focusing clearly on objects as they come closer to the eye.

LAZY EYE/amblyopia — the condition that results from the brain favoring the use of only one eye.

MIDDLE-AGED SIGHT/presbyopia — the difficulty middle-aged people have focusing clearly on near objects.

NEARSIGHTEDNESS/myopia — the difficulty of focusing clearly on objects as they get farther away.

OCCIPITAL LOBE/VISUAL CORTEX — the primary "seeing" center of the brain, located in the lower back of the head between your ears, where nerve impulses sent from the eyes are turned into visual images.

SACCADIC MOVEMENTS — the movements the eyes make as they scan their visual field at the rate of 60 to 70 times per second.

SUPPRESSION — the shutting off by the brain of an image or an impulse being presented to one eye in order to avoid confusion or discomfort.

TOP

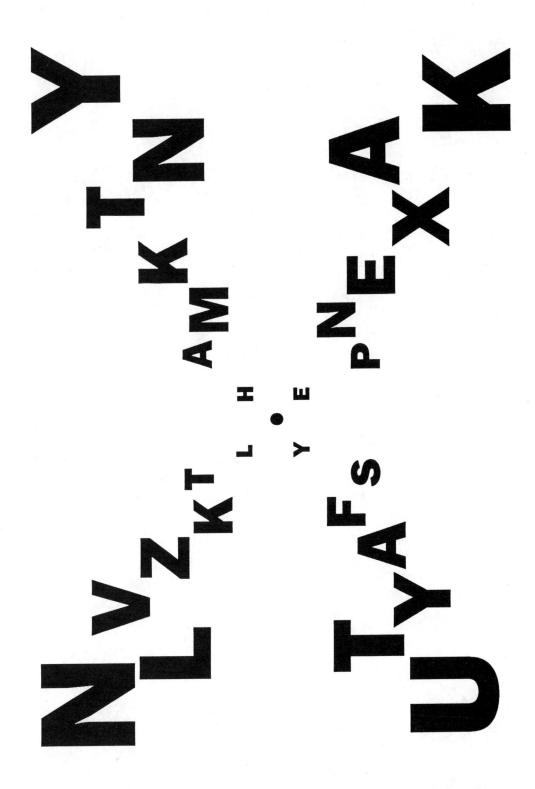

DOT CHART

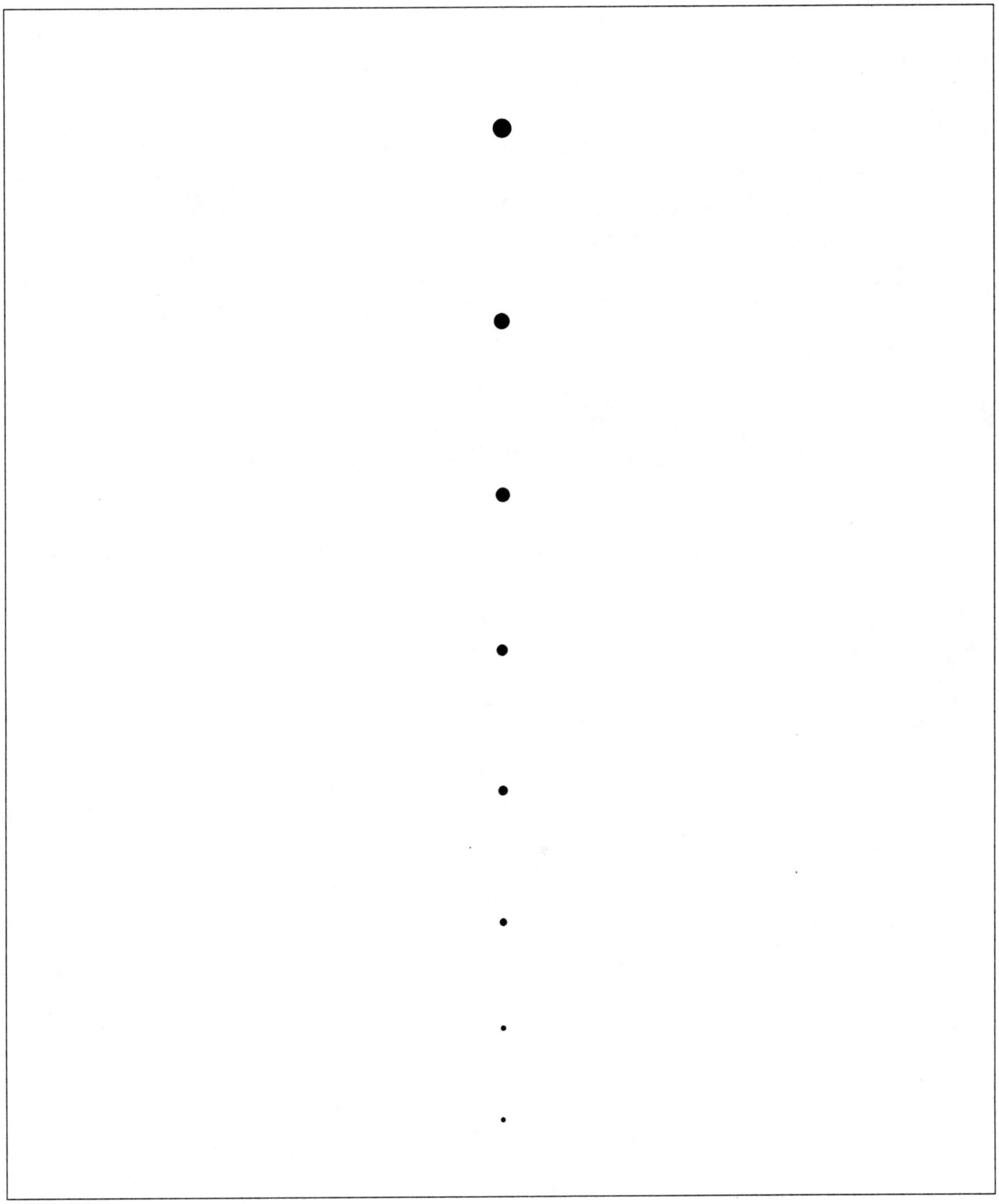

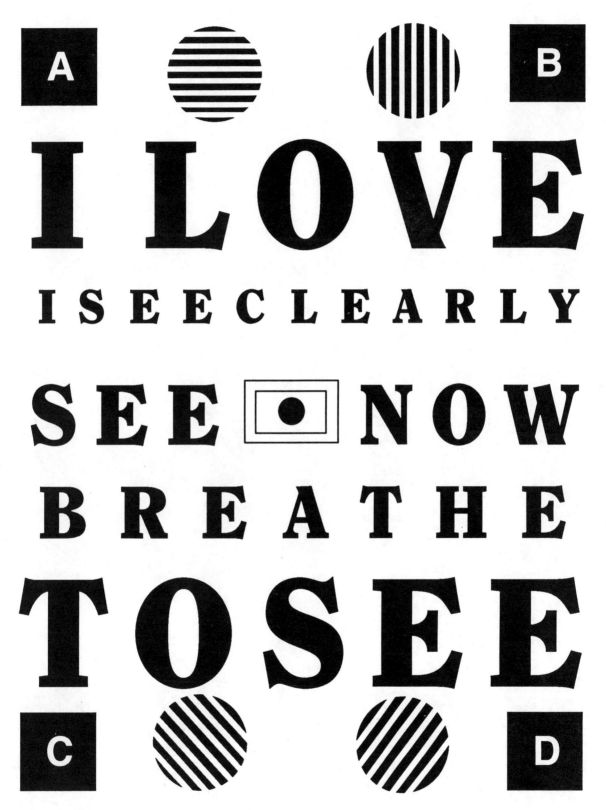

I can see more and more clearly

every day. The world is in sharp focus and it is easy for me to perform all tasks - including reading - easily and without any undue effort. I am letting go of all the unnecessary tension around my eyes. I am becoming more and more relaxed every day and I willingly receive everything positive that other people, and life, have to give me. I always acknowledge myself for all progress that I make and I am grateful for the support and encouragement given to me by my friends and family. I have all the discipline, desire and willingness that I need to reach my goal of having clear vision. As I regain my clearer vision, I am also regaining a feeling of health and youthfulness. I have all the vitality, enthusiasm and openness that I need to accomplish everything that is important to me and to receive the fruits of my labor. For this I am grateful.

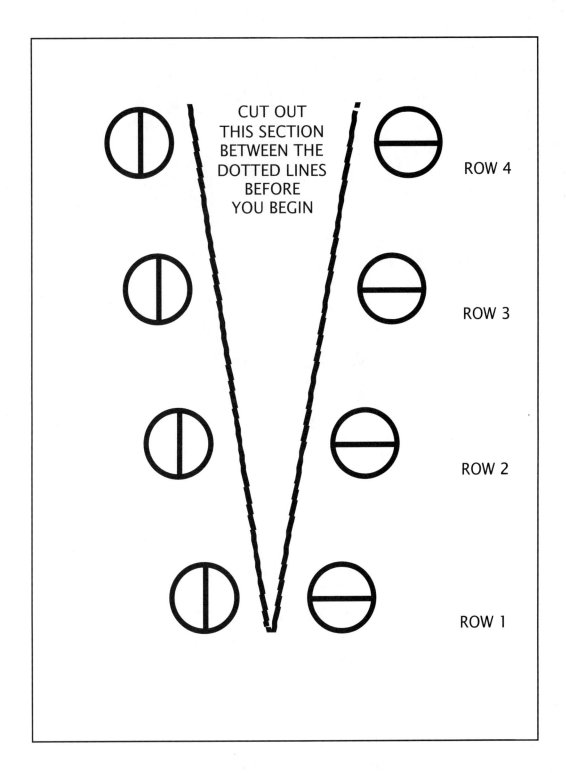

CUT OUT
THIS SECTION
BETWEEN THE
DOTTED LINES
BEFORE
YOU BEGIN

ROW 4

ROW 3

ROW 2

ROW 1

THE FIRST STAGE REPORT

The purpose of this report is twofold: 1) To assist the Cambridge Institute in updating, refining and modifying THE PROGRAM FOR BETTER VISION based on your comments and 2) To give you the opportunity to recap and review your own experience. Hopefully, this will bring to light insights and understandings that you may have overlooked or forgotten. **This report will be kept strictly confidential.**

Complete Part A before you begin and Parts B and C after you have completed THE FIRST STAGE. If you can, complete this report without using glasses or contacts. There are no right or wrong answers — only honest ones. Use additional paper if needed. After completing the report, remove (or copy) and mail to: Cambridge Institute, 65 Wenham, Topsfield MA 01983. We'll answer all questions that you ask.

_____	_____
Your Name	Date Started FIRST STAGE
_____	_____
Address	Date Completed FIRST STAGE
_____	_____ ____
City/State/Zip	Occupation Age
( ) _____	( ) _____
Day Phone	Eve Phone

PART A: COMPLETE BEFORE BEGINNING THE FIRST STAGE SCHEDULE

VISUAL HISTORY AND EVALUATION: This section asks you about your vision, attitudes, feelings and goals.

1. Describe your visual condition (nearsighted, farsighted, etc.).

2. What is your current prescription? (Write your most recent prescription if you have it.)

3. Approximately how many hours a day do you use your glasses/contacts?

4. Excluding glasses, have you had any medical treatment for your eyes (i.e., surgery or drugs)? If so, describe.

5. At what age did you begin using glasses or contact lenses?

6. Three things I like most about using glasses/contacts are

7. Three things I like least about using glasses/contacts are

8. Five activities that I regularly do without glasses/contacts (besides sleeping and bathing) are

9. Five activities I cannot or will not do without my glasses/contacts are

10. When I take my glasses/contacts off I feel

11. Three feelings I most closely associate with needing glasses/contacts are

12. Three feelings I most closely associate with not being able to see the world clearly are

13. Three positive feelings I would express more abundantly if my vision was clearer are

14. My three worst memories are

15. My three fondest memories are

16. I see the way that I do because

17. Three secret fears that I have about my vision are

18. Three major reasons I have for using The Program are

19. What would you like to achieve during the 8 weeks of THE FIRST STAGE?

20. Something else that I want to say about my vision is

PARTS B & C: COMPLETE AFTER FINISHING THE FIRST STAGE SCHEDULE

PROGRAM EXPERIENCE: This section asks you to reflect on your 8-week experience.

1. I now wear my glasses/contacts an average of _____ hours per day. Are you also using an under-corrected prescription?

2. Did you go to a behavioral optometrist at any time before, during and/or after THE FIRST STAGE? If so, what was the outcome of your visit(s)? If your progress was measured, what were the results?

3. How many days did it take you to complete the 8-week THE FIRST STAGE schedule?

4. Describe the changes in your eyesight that you've experienced. Be as specific as you can.

5. Describe any changes that you've noticed in your inner and emotional vision and in your attitudes.

6. Were there any turning points or major hurdles for you (physical, emotional, mental) during THE FIRST STAGE? Please describe.

7. Did you have any significant vision-related dreams during THE FIRST STAGE?

8. What did you learn about yourself?

9. What do you feel you've achieved?

10. The way that I feel about my vision now (compared to the way I used to feel) is

11. What surprised you the most about yourself during THE FIRST STAGE?

12. What specific techniques and visualizations do you plan to keep using?

13. How much time each day do you plan to practice?

14. Where would you like your vision to be eight weeks from today?

PROGRAM EVALUATION: This section asks you to evaluate this book.

1. How would you rate the following aspects: (Excellent, Good, Satisfactory, Fair)

   Ease of use _____

   Clarity of instructions _____

   Usefulness of information _____

   Overall effectiveness _____

2. Do you have any specific suggestions for improvement? Is there anything that you would change? Anything that you would exclude? Anything not there that you would want included?

3. Which week of THE FIRST STAGE did you find the most effective? ____ Why? Least effective? ____ Why?

4. Which week of THE FIRST STAGE did you find the hardest? _____ Why? The easiest? _____ Why?

5. At what point did you experience the greatest resistance? The greatest satisfaction?

6. Which technique or visualization did you enjoy or prefer the most? _____ Why?

The least? _____ Why?

7. Did you call the Institute for assistance? If so, what types of questions did you ask? Were you satisfied with the answers?

8. Any other comments?

9. Would you recommend this book to your friends? ___Yes___No. If not, why?

We'll send information about improving vision to these people that you suggest:

_____   _____
Name   Name

_____   _____
Address   Address

_____   _____
City/State/Zip   City/State/Zip

ADDITIONAL VISION CARE PRODUCTS

Here is a partial listing of the vision care items available from the Cambridge Institute. Some of these items are based on information from this book; others contain additional information and techniques. (Call or write for a current catalog.)

Audiotapes by Martin Sussman:

The six Vision Sessions from **THE FIRST STAGE** are available on 3 audiotapes. Many find that these audiotapes make practicing easier, more beneficial and more fun!

TAPE 1:   SIDE A: Fusion String Technique *(VISION SESSION 1: Pp. 64 - 68)*
SIDE B: Mind's Eye Visualization *(VISION SESSION 4: Pp. 90 - 92)*

TAPE 2:   SIDE A: Self Massage Techniques *(VISION SESSION 2: Pp. 69 - 78)*
SIDE B: Spectrum Visualization *(VISION SESSION 5: Pp. 93 - 96)*

TAPE 3:   SIDE A: Vision Chart Techniques *(VISION SESSION 3: Pp. 79 - 89)*
SIDE B: Memory Visualization *(VISION SESSION 6: Pp. 97 - 101)*

These techniques and visualizations from THE SECOND STAGE are also available:

TAPE 4:   LETTING GO OF VISUAL TENSION *(Pp. 135 - 138)*
TAPE 5:   PERIPHERAL AND FUSION AWARENESS *(Pp. 139 - 142)*
TAPE 6:   VISION AFFIRMATIONS *(Pp. 167 - 169)*
TAPE 7:   VISUAL AND MUSCULAR FLEXIBILITY *(Pp. 151 - 152)*

8. Eye Workout: *Gentle Routines of Eye Exercise and Body Relaxation*

This Eye Workout takes you through two different sessions of gentle head and neck stretches that allow you to release eye tension. The Eye Workout is especially helpful for nearsighted and farsighted people.

9. Forgiveness: *The Doorway to Emotional Clarity*

The subconscious memory of certain experiences — especially those that originate from around the time of the onset of a visual problem — is one of the major inner barriers that keep people from seeing clearly. This visualization will help you develop a more positive self-image, replacing negative feelings with self-love and clarity, leaving you more willing to see clearly.

10. LECTURE TAPE: What They Never Told You About Your Eyes

Mr. Sussman dispels the popular misconceptions about the causes of poor vision. You will learn how and why these vision problems can be improved using holistic methods. You'll also learn the "10 Keys to Better Vision" — simple visual habits that can protect your eyes throughout the day.

All audiotapes are $10.95 each

Also from Martin Sussman:

PHONE CONSULTATIONS and INDIVIDUALIZED TRAINING PROGRAMS: Talk with Martin Sussman about your vision. Let him answer all your questions and, if you are interested, he can design a schedule of practice that would work best for your eyes. Call the Cambridge Institute for more details.

Total Health at the Computer **by Martin Sussman and Dr. Ernest Loewenstein with Howard Sann:** This comprehensive guide shows you how to stay healthy, comfortable and productive at your computer. Called the *"best self-help book for computer users,"* **Total Health** gives you the Nine Fundamentals of Staying Healthy as well as easy-to-practice 3-minute routines to relieve the symptoms of Computer Stress Syndrome. You'll learn how to avoid glare, reduce exposure to electromagnetic radiation, save your eyesight and rid yourself of nagging body tension — headaches, backaches, shoulder, arm, wrist and hand tension. *$13.95*

Audiotapes by Dr. Gary Price Todd

Dr. Todd explains his approach to each of these medical problems. Dr. Todd's nutritional and metabolic treatment and the research supporting his methods are covered in greater depth and detail than in this book.

11. Cataract
12. Glaucoma
13. Macular Degeneration

All audiotapes are $10.95 each

Nutritional Supplements:

NUTRIPLEX FORMULA (developed by Dr. Gary Price Todd):

Vitamin A	10,000 IU	Magnesium	400 mg
Beta-Carotene (Vitamin A Activity)	10,000 IU	Potassium	50 mg
Vitamin D-3 (Fish Liver Oil)	200 IU	Iodine	150 mcg
Vitamin E (d-alpha Tocopheryl Succinate)	400 IU	Copper	2 mg
Vitamin K-1 (as Phytonadione)	60 mcg	Manganese	20 mg
Vitamin C (Ascorbic Acid Corn Free)	500 mg	Zinc	20 mg
Vitamin B-1 (Thiamine Mononitrate)	25 mg	Molybdenum	200 mcg
Vitamin B-2 (Riboflavin)	10 mg	Chromium GTF	200 mcg
Vitamin B-6 (Pyridoxine HCL)	25 mg	Selenium	200 mcg
Vitamin B-12 (on Ion Exchange Resin)	25 mcg	Vanadium	200 mcg
Niacin	50 mg	Boron	2 mg
Pantothenic Acid (d-Calcium Pantothenate)	150 mg	Methylsulfonylmethane	100 mg
Folic Acid	800 mcg	PABA	50 mg
Biotin	300 mcg	Citrus Bioflavinoids	200 mg
Choline (Bitartrate)	50 mg	Coenzyme Q-10	10 mg
Inositol	50 mg	Silica	40 mg
Calcium (Citrate)	200 mg		

30 day supply   **$24.99**   *60 day supply $45.99*

BILBERRY: If you suffer needlessly from night blindness, are sensitive to light or get "tired eyes" from extensive reading or computer use, bilberry is for you. Produced from bilberry extract (wild blueberries native to Europe and Asia) which contain anthocyanosides—instrumental in building healthy eyes. European studies indicate that bilberry may also be helpful for more serious eye problems such as glaucoma and macular degeneration.   *60 tablets $16.95*

GINGKO BILOBA: Gingko biloba supports blood flow to the eyes, improves concentration, memory and alertness. Has been used in Europe to aid in glaucoma and macular degeneration.   *60 tablets $16.95*

ORDER FORM FOR VISION CARE PRODUCTS

A new **Better Vision Catalog** will be sent with your order.

QUANTITY	ITEM NAME	COST	TOTAL
	SUB-TOTAL		
	Shipping and Handling		**4.95**
	Massachusetts residents add 5% State Sales Tax		
	TOTAL		

PAYMENT METHOD:
❏ Check   ❏ Money Order
❏ Credit Card: ❏ MasterCard ❏ Visa ❏ American Express

_____
credit card number

_____   _____
name on card   expiration date

SHIP TO: (Please print your name and address clearly)

_____
YOUR NAME

_____
ADDRESS

_____
CITY/STATE   ZIP

MAIL ORDERS TO:
Cambridge Institute ▪ 65 Wenham ▪ Topsfield MA 01983
CALL TOLL-FREE: 1-800-372-3937   **FAX ORDERS TO:** 978-887-3885

INDEX